THE MYSTERY OF GLAUCOMA

SOLVING WITH A DIFFERENT APPROACH

SYED SIKANDAR HASNAIN MD
General Ophthalmology
Porterville, California U.S.A.

THE MYSTERY OF GLAUCOMA
SOLVING WITH A DIFFERENT APPROACH

Copyright © 2018   Syed S. Hasnain MD
All Rights Reserved
Printed, May 2018

ISBN-10: 1732293406
ISBN-13: 978-1732293403

Dedicated to my parents for their great inspiration and to glaucoma patients as my service.

Preface

This book is about my hypothesis regarding the pathogenesis of primary open-angle glaucoma (POAG). It is not a substitute for a complete glaucoma textbook. POAG is chronic glaucoma also known simply as glaucoma.

Glaucoma is the leading cause of irreversible blindness in the world. It is estimated to affect between 70-80 million people worldwide. In chronic glaucoma there is a gradual, painless and irreversible loss of vision in normal quiet eyes. It is a serious condition since lost vision can't be regained. Since the visual loss is slow and gradual, glaucoma subjects usually don't seek medical attention unless there is a considerable loss of vision. Glaucoma is usually discovered during routine eye exams. Glaucoma is a very perplexing disease and despite extensive and ongoing research around the world, we still have no agreement on its pathogenesis.

Chronic glaucoma was given a separate entity in the 1850s. It was initially believed to be caused by elevated intraocular pressure (IOP). Statistically, the normal range of IOP is 10 to 21 mmHg. The IOP above 21mmHg or above is considered elevated IOP resulting in high-tension glaucoma (HTG). However, in the last few decades, glaucoma has been seen in subjects whose IOPs are consistently within the normal range. This is called normal-tension glaucoma (NTG).

This presents a puzzling question. Why is glaucoma also being caused by normal IOP? Both HTG and NTG have the same morphological features and a similar course of disease.

Why did I get involve in glaucoma research? In my early thirties, during my ophthalmology residency, I was found to have high IOP. It was around 30 mmHg in both eyes. All that was known at the time was that the elevated IOP would eventually cause glaucoma and blindness but not exactly how.

I had many unanswered questions about glaucoma but the most puzzling question: Why are the one million or so densely packed nerve fibers (NFs) in the optic nerve head (ONH) always being destroyed in an orderly sequence -from peripheral to central? This never occurs randomly.

If the NFs were being destroyed randomly, then we wouldn't be doing visual field tests in glaucoma. The reason we do visual field tests in glaucoma is because we are looking for predictable and pathognomonic visual field defects, or scotomas, in the paracentral area (10 to 20 degrees). These scotomas become more frequent and coalesce to become complete arcuate field defects as the glaucoma progresses. The arcuate field defects are a diagnostic feature of glaucoma as no other disease produces them.

However, the most salient feature of glaucoma is that the NFs are being destroyed in an orderly sequence starting with the most peripheral NFs and ending with the most central nerve fibers.

My puzzling question was that if the NFs are being destroyed in an orderly sequence, then we should expect the mechanism for their destruction to be an orderly one as well. The orderly loss of NFs can't be explained by any of the prevalent glaucoma theories such as the direct role of elevated IOP on the NFs, ischemia, neuro-degeneration, or apoptosis among many.

I was convinced that the orderly loss of NFs is perhaps the only lead we have in discovering the true pathogenesis of glaucoma. Surprisingly, no research had been done on this very distinctive feature of glaucoma. Not finding the answer for the orderly loss of NFs in literature and textbooks, I resorted to my own research.

My research led me to a hypothesis that the lamina cribrosa/optic disc may be sinking in its entirety. Due to sinking of the lamina cribrosa, the NFs are being stretched and severed starting with the most peripheral NFs and ending with the most central NFs at the scleral edge, in an orderly sequence. The sinking of the lamina cribrosa and severance of NFs can explain the orderly loss of NFs in glaucoma as explained in this book.

My article titled, "Scleral edge, not optic disc or retina is the primary site of injury in chronic glaucoma" describing the hypothesis was published in *Medical Hypotheses* in 2006.

The sinking optic disc and severance of NFs presents a paradigm shift to the current paradigm based on cupping of the optic disc and atrophy of NFs in glaucoma. This book will discuss in detail how I arrived at my hypothesis. This of course needs to be scientifically proven.

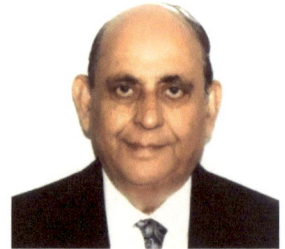

Syed S. Hasnain MD
General Ophthalmology
Porterville, California   United States
www.glaucomaparadigmshift.com

Foreward

Glaucoma is second to cataract amongst visual disabilities and it is a major cause of worldwide irreversible blindness. According to an authentic estimation there will be about 59 million people with open-angle glaucoma. Hence, it is extremely important to improve diagnosis and therapeutic approach to glaucoma. There are one million nerve fibers originating from the retinal ganglion cells (RGC) which leave the eye ball through the meshwork of lamina cribrosa to form the optic nerve.

In glaucoma there is an orderly destruction of nerve fibers from periphery to center (and not randomly) which is the foundation of perimetery. Now the whole mystery surrounds the orderly destruction of these nerve fibers. Many researchers have postulated various theories for the last 150 years regarding the pathogenesis of glaucoma *vis a vis* cupping of the disc. In fact, this is the crucial and important feature. The orderly destruction of nerve fibers cannot be ignored and be kept in sight otherwise any paradigm will be a redundant hypothesis. Recently, Prof. Marianne Shahsuvaryan Ph.D.,D.Sc., from Armenia, an exponent in the field of Glaucoma has convincingly propounded it to be a multifactorial and progressively neuro-degenerative disorder resulting in the death of axons of ganglion cells and lateral geniculate nuclei in the visual cortex resulting in optic atrophy, but the focal point of destruction of orderly nerve fibers still remains shrouded.

Dr. Syed Hasnain, a promising Pakistani researcher has spent his lifetime in searching the truth, has finally unveiled this mystery through his paradigm on scientific grounds. According to him, there is sinking of the disc in the scleral canal – a mechanical problem due to biological effect of raised IOP on the border tissue of Elschnig resulting in its degeneration. Sinking of the disc results in stretching and severance of nerve fibers at the scleral edge in an orderly sequence from peripheral to central. In fact, glaucoma is not an optic disc neuropathy, but an optic disc axotomy. Medicine is a subject which is constantly undergoing a proliferative change especially in the field of ophthalmology.

Dr. Hasnain has lucidly explained his paradigm, which the readers will find it very convincing in his book "The Mystery of Glaucoma". We are happy to know that scientists have readily accepted his paradigm and he deserves our heartfelt commendations for unveiling this mystery. We recommend this book to the budding ophthalmologists and practicing glaucoma specialists to accept his innovative paradigm with open heart.

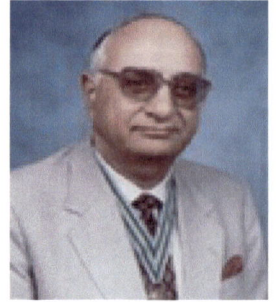

Prof. M. Yasin Khan Durrani
FRCOphth (Lond)
Former: Professor of Ophthalmology
Rawalpindi Medical University & Chief Editor
Ophthalmology Update, Islamabad. Pakistan
www.ophthalmologyupdate.com

Contents

Chapter 1

What is Glaucoma?

The term glaucoma goes back to Hippocratic times. It was described as the blindness associated with greenish/bluish haze in the pupil of the eye. Initially, both terms cataract and glaucoma were indistinguishable and were used to describe blind eyes until 1700 A.D. Afterwards, cataract was identified as a disease of the lens and its blindness was curable and reversible. Whereas, glaucoma was associated with increased intraocular pressure (IOP) and its blindness as being permanent and irreversible.

What is intraocular pressure? The eyeball is a closed organ which contains fluid known as aqueous humor which provides oxygen and nutrients to the intraocular structures of the eye. This fluid is continuously being formed and replaced after giving nutrition to the eye. While this fluid is within the closed eyeball, it creates pressure known as intraocular pressure (IOP). The IOP exerts pressure on the wall of the eyeball including the optic nerve head (ONH) containing all the nerve fibers (NFs) as they exit the eyeball on their way to the brain.

In the beginning, all glaucomatous eyes were believed to be inflamed, painful with increased IOP until another category of glaucoma surfaced in the 1850s in which the eyes were white and painless but having increased intraocular pressure.

A breakthrough in ophthalmology occurred in 1851 with the invention of the ophthalmoscope by Hermann von Helmholtz. This enabled us to view the optic discs of subjects with painless and quiet blind eyes with increased IOP. The optic discs of these patients were found to be depressed rather than being normally flat. In 1856, Heinrich Muller, a pathologist, named these depressed discs as cupped discs. These cupped discs were thought to be due to the direct effect of increased IOP (Figure 1).

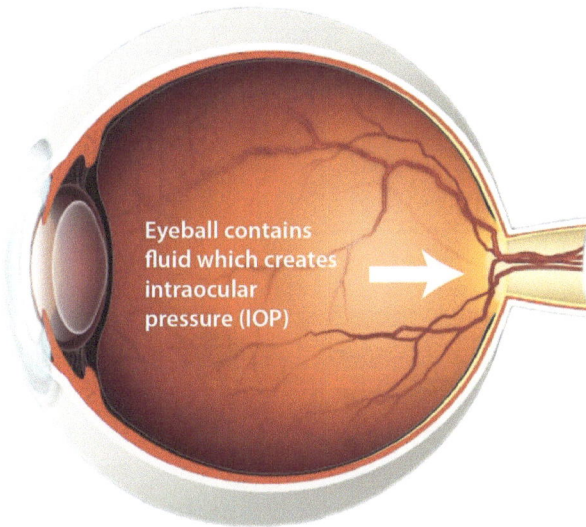

Eyeball contains
fluid which creates
intraocular
pressure (IOP)

Figure 1. Schematic Diagram. A closed eyeball contains clear fluid which creates intraocular pressure. Normal IOP is 10 to 21mmHg. If the IOP becomes elevated, it will damage the optic disc resulting in glaucoma and irreversible blindness.

Donders (1862) described this type of glaucoma as simple glaucoma. The term simple implied that the eyes were simply white and painless. Currently, simple glaucoma is called primary open-angle glaucoma (POAG) or chronic glaucoma or simply as glaucoma. POAG is the most common type of glaucoma and is under discussion in this book. This book does not discuss other kinds of glaucoma such as acute and closed-angle glaucomas.

Over the past 160 years, the term cupping has become synonymous with glaucoma. In the past, chronic glaucoma was always believed to be associated with increased intraocular pressure and cupping was thought to be due to the direct effect of elevated intraocular pressure. However, after the invention of the Goldmann applanation tonometer in the 1950s, the measurement of IOP became more precise and accurate.

We found that many chronic glaucoma patients had their IOPs consistently within the normal range (10 to 21mmHg). Therefore, those subjects having all the features of chronic glaucoma but with normal range IOPs were classified as having normal-tension glaucoma (NTG). Those subjects with IOP of 21 mmHg or above were classified as those with high-tension glaucoma (HTG).

It is believed HTG and NTG are equally divided in the general population. However, in certain races such as the Japanese, NTG is more common. The NTG is also more common in patients with poor systemic problems such as chronic hypotension, COPD, sleep apnea, long-term smokers and those with high myopia. Since high myopia is more common in Japanese, this may be the reason for increased prevalence of NTG in Japanese.

Some researchers think of NTG as a separate entity, but HTG and NTG have the same glaucomatous features and course of disease. I believe that since HTG is caused by elevated IOP, NTG must be caused by even normal IOP but acting as elevated IOP in that particular subject. Both HTG and NTG will lead to a common ground of injury which we will discuss later.

What is the definition of glaucoma?

We don't have consensus on a definition for glaucoma, which keeps on changing. The 2015 edition of the American Academy of Ophthalmology defined POAG as:

"a chronic progressive optic neuropathy in adults in which there is characteristic acquired atrophy of the optic nerve and loss of the retinal ganglion cells and their axons. This condition is associated with an open anterior chamber angle by gonioscopy."

The aforementioned definition of glaucoma has neither taken into account the role of IOP nor the characteristic visual field loss. Instead, it has focused mainly on the optic neuropathy and the loss of retinal ganglion cells.

My position argues against glaucoma being an optic neuropathy. These arguments are mainly based on the main distinctive feature of glaucoma – the orderly loss of NFs corroborating with visual field defects. This will be discussed later in the book.

Chapter 2

The Visual Pathways and Blood Supply

It is imperative to become familiar with the arrangement of NFs in the retina and in the ONH and their blood supply. They are very important in understanding the pathogenesis of glaucoma and the production of glaucomatous visual field defects.

The one million or so nerve fibers in the retina are arranged in layers, superficial (closest to vitreous) to deep (closest to sclera). The NFs originating closest to the optic disc lie most superficial and exit from the most central part of the ONH. In contrast, the most peripheral NFs originate from the most distant part of the retina or farthest from the ONH, lie deepest (closest to sclera) and exit closest to the edge of the scleral opening (Figure 2).

The NFs originating from the nasal retina proceed directly to the nasal part of the optic disc. However, the situation is different in the temporal retina due to presence of the macular fibers. The NFs originating from the nasal aspect of the macular area proceed directly to the temporal part of the disc.

The NFs originating from the temporal macular and temporal retina arch above and below the macular fibers to reach the superior and inferior poles of the ONH respectively. These are known as the arcuate nerve fibers.

Although the arcuate NFs have become separated from the rest of the NFs, they are still lying in layers from superficial to deep as do the macular and rest of the NFs (Figure 3).

The arrangement of NFs as they come from the retina is the same in the prelaminar and laminar part of the ONH. However, in the retrolaminar region, the macular fibers become centrally placed in the optic nerve. In the optic chiasma, the nasal half of the fibers cross to the opposite side and form the optic tract until they synapse in the lateral geniculate nucleus (LGN). From the LGN, the optic radiation begins and extends to the occipital cortex.

Blood Circulation of the Optic Disc

The optic disc has a dual blood supply - retinal and ciliary circulation.

Retinal Circulation: the central retinal artery (CRA) is a branch of the ophthalmic artery but it is mainly destined for the retina, though on its way it gives some contribution to the retrolaminar region and superficial nerve fiber layer of the ONH.

Ciliary Circulation: the ophthalmic artery, a branch of the internal carotid also gives origin to two posterior ciliary arteries which divide into short posterior ciliary arteries (SPCAs). Some of them form the arterial circle of Zinn-Haller which supplies the prelaminar, laminar and the border tissue of Elschnig (BT). Sometimes this arterial circle is not present or is incomplete in which case the branches from SPCAs supply this region directly (Figure 4).

The CRA is a higher pressure system (around 60 mmHg) compared to the ciliary circulation since it remains solitary from its origin from the ophthalmic artery until its emergence at the central part of the optic disc. The ciliary circulation is of lower pressure (around 25 mmHg) due to its multiple branches.

The important point to remember is that the border tissue of Elschnig is exclusively supplied by ciliary circulation and does not receive any contribution from the CRA at all (Hayreh, 1970). This fact will be very important in the pathogenesis of glaucoma as we will discuss later.

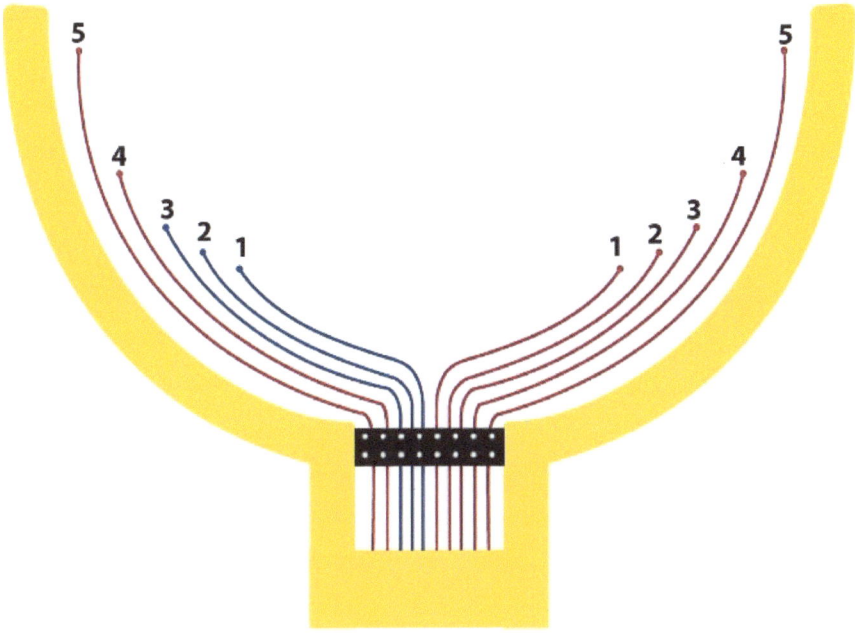

Figure 2. Schematic Diagram. Arrangement of nerve fibers in the retina and optic disc. The most peripheral fibers (5) originate farthest from the optic disc, lie deepest (closest to the sclera) and exit nearest to the scleral edge. The most central fibers (1) originate closest to the disc, lie most superficial (closest to vitreous) and exit from the most central part of the disc.

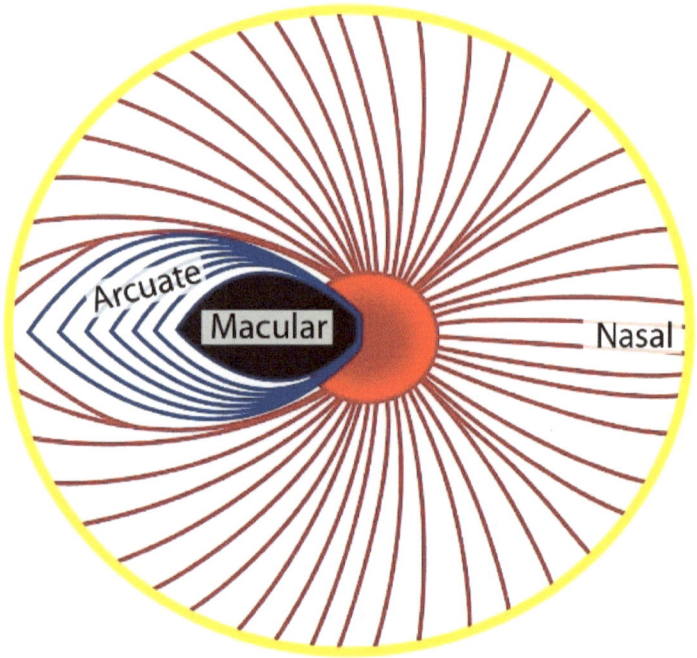

Figure 3. Schematic Diagram. Arrangement of nerve fibers in the retina and optic disc. The arcuate fibers arch above and below the macular fibers to reach the poles of the optic disc.

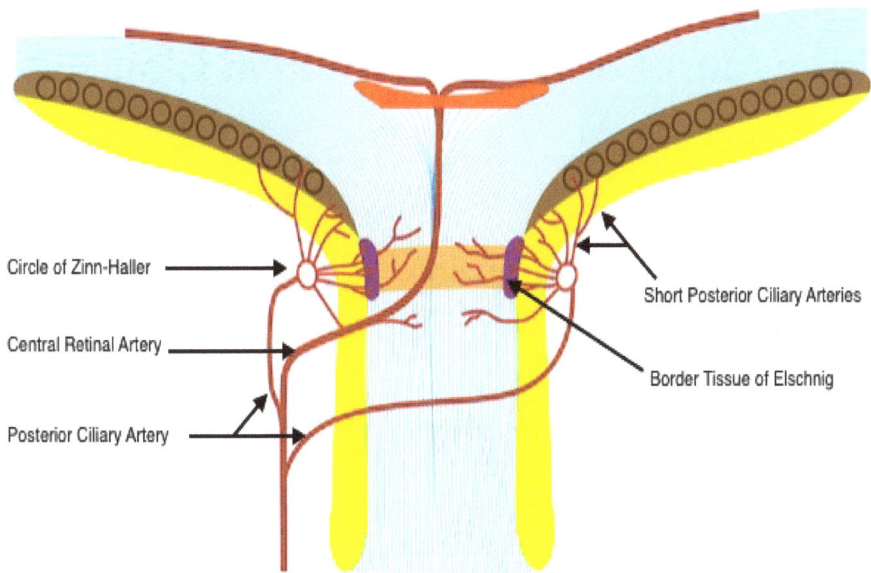

**Figure 4. Schematic Diagram. Blood supply of the optic disc.
The central retinal artery (CRA) is destined for the retina. Short
posterior ciliary arteries form the circle of Zinn-Haller, supply
the LC and border tissue of Elschnig (BT). Note: The CRA does
not contribute to the BT.**

Chapter 3

The Most Puzzling Question in Glaucoma

The most puzzling question of glaucoma, which is rarely discussed: Why are the one million or so densely packed NFs in the optic nerve head are always being destroyed in an orderly tandem sequence, one-by-one, from peripheral to central? They are never destroyed randomly.

The orderly and predictable visual field loss is the reason we do visual field tests in glaucoma. Otherwise, the role of perimetry would be meaningless. The orderly loss of NFs is perhaps the only lead we have in discovering the correct pathogenesis of glaucoma. Unfortunately, this issue has never been adequately addressed.

What is the Orderly Loss of NFs in glaucoma?

The orderly loss of visual fields in glaucoma is corroborated by the arrangement of NFs in the optic disc. The most peripheral 360 degrees of NFs are destroyed first in glaucoma resulting in generalized constriction of the peripheral visual field. However the peripheral visual field loss has little diagnostic value in glaucoma due to normal variation of the limits of the peripheral field. Moreover, other diseases like cataract can also produce peripheral field constriction.

While the generalized peripheral field constriction is occurring, the isolated scotomas are being produced in the 10-20 degrees of the paracentral area belonging to the superior and inferior arcuate fibers. These small isolated scotomas are being produced due to destruction of the arcuate fibers, singly or in small numbers.

As more of the arcuate fibers are destroyed, the isolated scotomas become enlarged and more frequent which eventually coalesce to become complete superior and inferior arcuate scotomas.

When the entire arcuate fibers are destroyed and depleted, the sharply defined superior and inferior arcuate scotomas are produced. When joined together, they become a ring scotoma with a characteristic nasal step, which is a pathognomonic and unique feature of glaucomatous field defects as no other optic disc disease produces them.

Arcuate scotomas with the nasal step fully corroborate with the arrangement of NFs in the ONH. Therefore, the NFs are being destroyed either in the prelaminar or laminar region of the ONH which we will discuss later. Moreover, glaucomatous field loss corroborating with the arrangement of NFs in the ONH suggests that the pathology lies in the axons, not in the soma of retinal ganglion cells (RGC).

Although the arcuate scotomas in glaucoma were discovered in 1890s by Jannik Bjerrum and then confirmed by his pupil Ronnie, we still don't have any agreement as to the cause of their production. As glaucoma progresses, the peripheral field constriction also advances and joins the superior and inferior arcuate scotomas ultimately leaving about 10 degrees of central vision which is also lost at the end-stage. The orderly loss of NFs is well corroborated with the arrangement of NFs in the ONH and also with the visual field defects in glaucoma.

This presents a puzzling question. If the NFs are being destroyed in an orderly sequence in glaucoma, then the mechanism for their destruction should be an orderly one as well. We have to find that mechanism.

In Chapter 4, we will evaluate the prevalent glaucoma theories and whether they can answer the orderly loss of NFs which is characteristic of this disease. For any glaucoma theory to prevail, it must also demonstrate and prove the orderly loss of NFs. Otherwise it would be of no value.

Chapter 4

Prevalent Glaucoma Theories Versus The Orderly Loss of Nerve Fibers

In the forthcoming discussion, we will analyze the prevalent glaucoma theories in the context of the orderly loss of nerve fibers. However, before we discuss this important feature, it is imperative to review the historical background of the cupping concept.

The Cupping Paradigm

After the invention of the ophthalmoscope in 1851 by Hermann von Helmholtz, ophthalmologists for the first time were able to see the optic discs of chronic glaucoma patients (called at that time, simple glaucoma) and found that their optic disc had become cupped instead of being normally flat. They were most likely observing the end-stage glaucomatous discs of simple glaucoma subjects.

The term 'cupping' was given in 1856 by Heinrich Muller, an ophthalmic pathologist (Duke-Elder, 1969). During that time, majority of ophthalmologists agreed with the phenomenon of cupping or the cupped shaped depression of the optic disc, which they thought was due to the direct effect of elevated IOP on the normally flat optic disc.

But there was one dissenter. Dr. James Dixon disagreed that cupping was due to the direct effect of elevated IOP. Dixon argued that if the mechanical force of elevated IOP was strong enough to cause cupping, or depression of the optic disc, then that same strong force should have also displaced the lens and iris forward. However, Dixon's arguments were rejected by a prominent ophthalmologist, Sir William Bowman, in favor of cupping. Thereafter, the concept of cupping survived.

After this, no one seemed to have challenged the concept of cupping. Unfortunately, a wrong cupping paradigm was born which is still flourishing until this day and has become synonymous with glaucoma.

With due respect, the ophthalmologists of the 1850s were correct in assuming that the optic discs of chronic glaucoma subjects had become cupped due to the direct force of elevated IOP. It was their reasonable assumption at the time that the mechanical force of elevated IOP had transformed the normally flat disc into a glaucomatous cupped disc. Moreover, the ophthalmology field was in its infancy at the time and ophthalmoscopes were rudimentary. Candlelight was used to illuminate the fundus as there was no electricity at that time.

As time progressed, the cupping paradigm became more deeply embedded in glaucoma. Nearly over a century later in the 1960s, instead of rejecting the cupping paradigm, we introduced the term cup-to-disc ratio for the diagnosis and monitoring of glaucoma progression (Armaly, 1969).
It was assumed that in glaucoma, physiological cups (the original optic cups of birth) begin enlarging concentrically and thus become pathological or glaucomatous cups due to direct mechanical force of elevated IOP.

My belief is that ophthalmologists of the 1850s had no conception of physiological cups when the term cupping was given. As time passed and ophthalmoscopes improved, ophthalmologists started noticing physiological cups of various sizes and theorized that they were enlarging in glaucoma. Thus, researchers assumed that if someone was born with a large physiological cup such as 0.6, that subject would take less time to become 100% pathologically cupped or become totally blind compared to someone born with a small cup such as 0.2.

This was probably the reason that the concept of cup-to-disc ratio was introduced giving further credence to the cupping paradigm and thus great importance to the size of physio-logical cups in the pathogenesis of glaucoma. Unfortunately, the cup-to-disc ratio has become an established standard in the screening, diagnosis and monitoring of glaucoma progression. Today, we cannot describe the stages of glaucomatous discs without mentioning their cup-to-disc ratio.

Ironically, we are using the same parameter of cupping in describing both physiological as well as glaucomatous cupping. This big mistake has created a conundrum in the diagnosis of glaucoma. Subjects born with large physiological cups but with normal IOP are being treated as normal-tension glaucoma or glaucoma-suspect. However, subjects born with small or no physiological cups, even with elevated IOP, are ignored treatment as having ocular hypertension.

Surprisingly, this is considered as a benign condition even with elevated IOP. Since the size of the optic cup has become very important in the diagnosis of glaucoma, ophthal-mologists are faced with an even bigger dilemma - how to differentiate between a large physiological cup and glauco-matous cup for which we still don't have any proper standard for differentiation.

It is our great mistake to use the term cupping in describing both physiological as well as glaucomatous cupping. We have never seen such a mistake of using the same parameter in describing both the physiological and the diseased state of an organ in other branches of medicine. Similarly, we don't have terms such as normal hypertension or benign high blood pressure.

What are the Physiological Cups?

The physiological cups are produced by varying degrees of atrophy of the Bergmeister's papilla - a tuft of blood vessels which supplies nutrition to the lens in fetal life (Wolff, 1968). Physiological cups are fibrous tissue remnants of Bergmeister's papilla, sometimes as large as covering 90% of the disc surface, termed as a 0.9 cup-to-disc ratio. If there is no remnant tissue, then there would be no physiological cup and such an optic disc would be described as having a 0.0 cup-to-disc ratio (Figures 5,6).

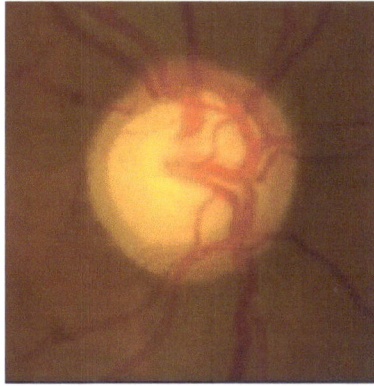
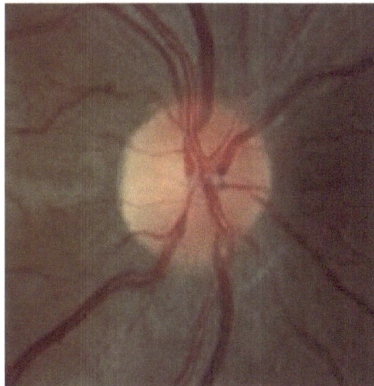

Figure 5. A. Physiological cup of 0.8   B. Physiological cup of 0.0.

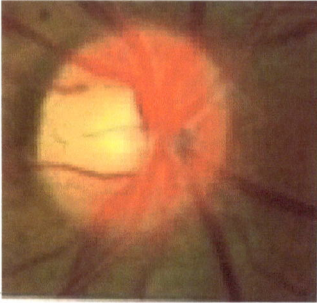

Physiological cup 0.2

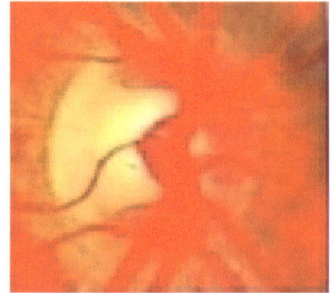

Physiological cup 0.4

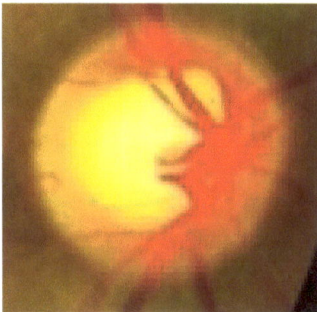

Physiological cup 0.6

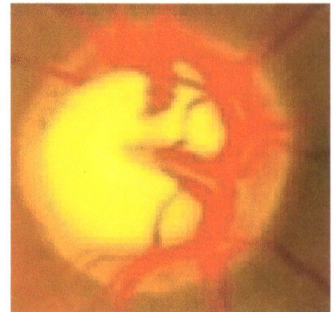

Physiological cup 0.8

Figure 6. Features of physiological cups. The entire 360 degrees of the rim area is of uniform reddish color. The margins of the cup are well defined. There is no break or notching in the cup margin and no nasal shifting of central vessels. Normal vision and no field defects.

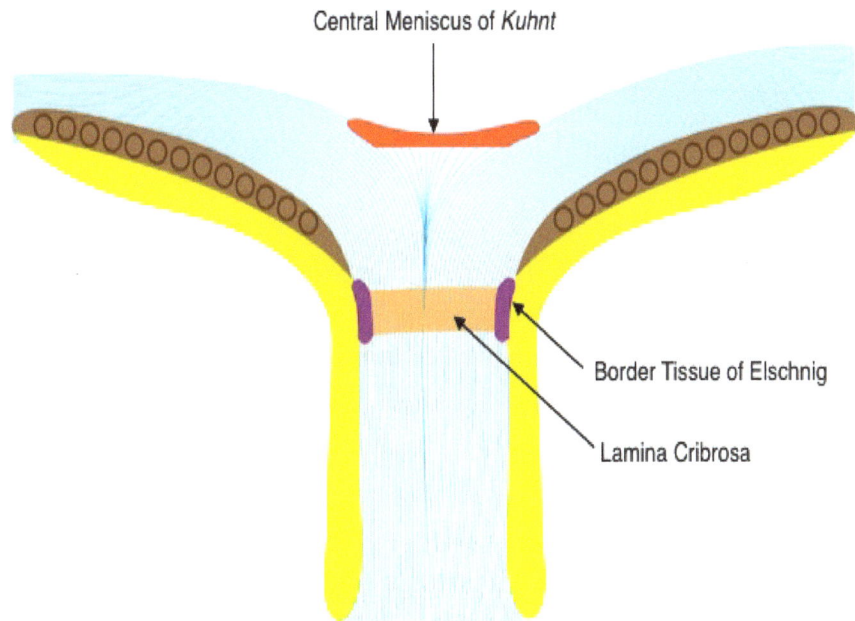

Figure 7. Schematic Diagram. Anatomy of the optic disc. The red area is the central meniscus of *Kuhnt,* remnant of Bergmeister's papilla. The purple area on each side of the lamina cribrosa is the border tissue of Elschnig.

In summary, the base of the physiological cup determines the size of whether an individual has a cup-to-disc ratio of 0.2 or 0.9. However, the physiological cup is nothing more than a fibrous tissue remnant of fetal life. In the histology of the normal disc, this remnant tissue is identified as the central meniscus of *Kuhnt* lying superficially on the surface of the optic disc densely packed with NFs. In other words, the NFs are present underneath this meniscus or so-called cupped area as well (Figure 7).

Is the optic disc really an analogue to a doughnut?

It is widely mentioned that the entire NFs of the disc are present in the so-called neuroretinal rim, while the central cup area is an empty hole devoid of nerve fibers – an analogue to a doughnut. This would imply that if someone is born with a physiological cup of 0.8, then 80% of the central area would be a hole devoid of NFs. In other words, the entire NFs are present only in the remaining 20% of the disc area or in the so-called neuroretinal rim.

It is a fallacy to describe the arrangement of NFs in the optic disc as an analogue to a doughnut. There is not a single histology available depicting a doughnut-shaped configuration of NFs in any disc, glaucomatous or otherwise. The lamina cribrosa (LC) of every optic disc is densely packed with NFs all the way to the center of the LC. There is hardly any vacant space except for the central retinal vessels.

If the optic disc indeed were doughnut-shaped, then the discs having larger cups or in other words, larger holes, should be less prone to glaucoma since the force of IOP would be rapidly dissipated in larger holes - the neuroretinal rim would escape injury.

The larger the hole, the less likely there would be injury to the neuroretinal rim. If the optic disc is an analogue to a doughnut, then how can a holed LC also become posteriorly bowed at all? When 360 degrees of prelaminar retinal nerve fibers converge in the optic disc, a small dimple is produced in the central part of the disc. But this is not what we define as cupping.

The concept of the physiological cup and neuroretinal rim, being an analogue to a doughnut has no histological proof. Since physiological cups are not doughnut-shaped, the concept of cupping, cup-to-disc ratio and the neuroretinal rim become redundant.

The current definition of glaucomatous cupping

There are two definitions of glaucomatous cupping. The first definition, when the physiological cups starts enlarging concentrically due to elevated IOP and becomes glaucomatously cupped. The second definition, when the lamina cribrosa starts bowing posteriorly or becomes cupped due to the mechanical force of elevated IOP.

Both definitions are contradictory since one definition implies the concentric enlargement of the physiological cup and the other as posterior bowing of the lamina cribrosa. Ironically, we talk much about cupping yet we have no clear conception of the phenomenon of cupping. In some of today's research, the depth of the glaucomatous cup is defined as the distance between the opening of Bruch's membrane and the anterior prelaminar neural surface. Thereby, disregarding the lamina cribrosa as part of cupping.

It is hard to comprehend that the multilayered connective tissue plate of the LC is so delicate and flimsy that it will start bowing posteriorly with a rise of about 10 mmHg of IOP, yet not bow in cases of acute glaucoma when the IOP becomes extremely elevated. We don't observe acute cupping occurring in acute glaucoma. There is no histological evidence of posterior bowing of the lamina cribrosa.

Can cupping result in the orderly loss of NFs in glaucoma?

If cupping was indeed taking place, then the most superficial (closest to the vitreous) and most central fibers of the ONH would had been destroyed first. This would have resulted, first in concentric enlargement of the blind spot followed by loss of macular fibers or immediate loss of central vision. But in actuality, the opposite is occurring in glaucoma. The peripheral fibers are destroyed first and central fibers last until the end-stage of glaucoma.

The glaucomatous field defects do not corroborate with the concept of cupping. The cupping paradigm cannot explain the orderly loss of NFs from peripheral to central. Most importantly, since cupping cannot explain the orderly production of glaucomatous field defects from peripheral to central, it must not be occurring at all in glaucoma. If cupping is not occurring then what may be happening? We will discuss this later.

Can elevated IOP acting directly result in the orderly loss of NFs in glaucoma?

It is inconceivable that elevated IOP acting directly on the one million or so densely packed NFs could result in their, one-by-one, orderly destruction. We have ruled out the role of elevated IOP by inducement of cupping in the production of the orderly loss of NFs in glaucoma. Despite the many schematic pictures in textbooks showing elevated IOP directly damaging the optic disc, IOP acting directly on the NFs can't result in their orderly loss. However, it is an established fact that elevated IOP is the cause of glaucoma. But, the elevated IOP cannot directly cause the orderly loss of NFs. There must be some indirect way in which elevated IOP is causing the orderly loss of NFs in glaucoma.

Can direct ischemia result in the orderly loss of NFs in glaucoma?

It is proposed that elevated IOP compresses the capillaries supplying the NFs resulting in ischemia and their eventual death. It has been mentioned that the radial peripapillary capillaries supplying the arcuate fibers are unusually susceptible to elevated IOP, resulting in ischemia and the death of arcuate fibers (Henkind, 1967). Direct ischemic injury cannot explain the one-by-one, orderly loss of NFs in glaucoma from peripheral to central.

There is always the production of very few isolated scotomas in the paracentral area in the initial stages of glaucoma which become more frequent and enlarged. They ultimately coalesce to form a complete arcuate scotoma. Initial isolated scotomas suggest that NFs are dying individually or in very small numbers in the early stages of glaucoma. However, as glaucoma progresses, all the arcuate nerve fibers are eventually destroyed. If ischemia was a factor, then all the arcuate NFs should have been destroyed at once. Not one-by-one at a time. Moreover, the arcuate field defects have sharply defined margins that couldn't be produced by any ischemic insult.

If capillaries are becoming occluded due to elevated IOP, then how can we explain their occlusion due to normal IOP in normal-tension glaucoma?

It has been theorized that the blood supply to the axons in the laminar region is impeded by distortion of the laminar beams due to posterior bowing of the LC, resulting in ischemia. This implicates the lamina cribrosa as the site of injury in glaucoma, but the LC couldn't be the site of injury based on the orderly loss of NFs in glaucoma.

Thus, direct ischemia of the NFs cannot result in the orderly loss of NFs in glaucoma. However, I believe ischemia is playing a very important, but indirect role, in the orderly destruction of NFs in glaucoma. This we will discuss later.

Can neurodegeneration result in the orderly loss of NFs in glaucoma?

Glaucoma is also theorized as a neurodegenerative disease akin to Parkinson's and Alzheimer's Disease. My belief is that glaucoma is thought of as a neuro- degenerative or brain disease, because of the simultaneous death of RGCs, neurons of the lateral geniculate nucleus (LGN) and of the visual cortex. It is theorized that glaucoma starts with the death of RGCs, triggered by elevated IOP, leading to the death of neurons of the LGN and of the visual cortex.

It is hard to conceive that once triggered by elevated IOP, neurodegeneration of RGCs would be so precise and systematic that it will always begin with the RGCs serving the peripheral vision and end with the RGCs serving the central vision in an orderly sequence. This would be very unlikely. The random degeneration of the neurons is the hallmark of a

neurodegenerative disease. The course of a neurodegenerative disease varies in each individual. Therefore, in
view of the orderly loss of NFs, glaucoma cannot be a
neurodegenerative disease.

Can apoptosis result in the orderly loss of NFs in glaucoma?

It is also theorized that elevated IOP triggers the apoptosis
(suicide) of the retinal ganglion cells (RGC) and thus initiates
glaucoma. Apoptosis or self-destruction of cells always occurs
randomly - never in an orderly sequence.

For apoptosis to occur in glaucoma, our genes would have to
be smart enough to first predict the impending glaucoma so
that the RGCs would then initiate apoptosis or start
committing suicide in an orderly sequence, starting with those
serving the peripheral vision and ending with those RGCs
which serve the central vision - a very unlikely scenario.

Apoptosis is a genetically regulated form of cell death to get
rid of overproduced cells in intrauterine development, or get
rid of diseased cells after birth, but not the normal cells. Why
should apoptosis occur in healthy RGCs? In glaucoma,
normal healthy RGCs are being destroyed in an orderly
sequence, which would be out of the scope of apoptosis.

Moreover, apoptosis is genetically regulated. So why are the
RGCs dying in an orderly sequence in traumatic glaucoma
which is not genetically controlled? In view of the orderly
and systematic loss of NFs, it would be inconceivable that
glaucoma is due to apoptosis of the RGCs.

Can low cerebrospinal fluid pressure result in the orderly loss of NFs in glaucoma?

Recently, theories have been postulated that glaucoma is due to low cerebrospinal fluid (CSF) pressure. It is stated that the lamina cribrosa separates the CSF pressure and IOP. Due to lower CSF pressure, elevated IOP will cause posterior bowing of the LC. In other words, induce cupping. Conversely if CSF pressure is higher than IOP, the LC will bow anteriorly.

It is inconceivable that the multilayered connective tissue of the lamina cribrosa, densely packed with NFs is so flimsy that it will move back and forth with a small change in pressure difference between CSF pressure and IOP. The normal CSF pressure is around 8-15 mmHg, therefore every subject having an IOP above 15 mmHg should show signs of posterior bowing of the LC. In this scenario we should be seeing a lot more glaucomas than the currently estimated 2% of the general population.

If the multilayered rigid LC is indeed so flimsy, then we should have seen acute cupping occurring in acute glaucoma where the IOP becomes extremely elevated to 60 mmHg or more. But there is no acute cupping occurring in acute glaucoma.

It is theorized that low CSF pressure causes glaucoma by the cupping scenario, which we have already refuted. Since cupping can't result in the orderly destruction of NFs in glaucoma, the CSF pressure appears to have no role in glaucoma.

Then, why are NFs being destroyed in an orderly sequence in glaucoma?

My argument so far is that elevated IOP acting directly or by direct ischemia could not result in the orderly loss of NFs. Also, elevated IOP either by inducing cupping, posterior bowing of the LC, neurodegeneration, apoptosis or any other biological mechanism couldn't result in the orderly loss of NFs. This is for sure.

Therefore, all glaucoma theories postulating the direct role of elevated IOP on the RGCs or on their axons, whether in the retina or in the lamina cribrosa become invalid. None of them can explain the orderly and systematic loss of NFs in glaucoma.

Nevertheless, without any doubt, it is an established fact that elevated IOP is the definitive cause of glaucoma. For example, in the case of unilateral traumatic glaucoma, the moderately elevated IOP is the only factor present in a healthy subject - one who never got treatment due to lack of symptoms. The occurrence of unilateral traumatic glaucoma proves that elevated IOP alone can result in glaucoma without taking into account any additional contributory factors

This presents a puzzling question. If glaucoma is definitively caused by elevated IOP, but at the same time elevated IOP acting directly on the NFs couldn't result in their orderly loss, then how are the NFs being destroyed in an orderly and systematic sequence? How do we solve this dilemma?

If elevated IOP acting directly on the NFs couldn't result in their orderly loss, then there must be some indirect mechanical way to explain the orderly loss of NFs. Even if that mechanical scenario may have resulted from the biological effect of elevated IOP on some important component of the optic disc.

What may be that mechanical scenario?

Chapter 5

Glaucoma: A Two-Stage Disease

Since elevated IOP can't result in the orderly loss of NF's by its direct action, some indirect mechanism may be occurring. It is hypothesized that glaucoma is a two-stage disease. The first, a biological stage, followed by a second mechanical stage.

In the biological stage, there is degeneration of the border tissue of Elschnig (BT) due to chronic ischemia resulting from the subacute and chronic compression of border tissue circulation - by elevated IOP or even by normal IOP acting as elevated IOP in that particular subject.

The biological stage is latent and pre-perimetric glaucoma. The circular BT keeps the LC firmly in place in the scleral opening (Figure 8). Therefore, degeneration of the BT would result in loosening and sinking of the lamina cribrosa; leading to initiation of the mechanical stage or perimetric glaucoma.

During the mechanical stage, the lamina cribrosa starts sinking in the scleral canal. As a result, the NFs are stretched as one end is attached to the soma of the RGC and the other end entangled in bundles in the pores of the LC. The NFs would ultimately break at the scleral edge. They become severed starting with the most peripheral NFs, being closest to the scleral edge, and ending with the most central in an orderly tandem sequence.

The First Stage: Degeneration of the Border Tissue

Why would the border tissue degenerate? The eyeball is supplied by dual circulation through the ciliary and central retinal artery (CRA). The border tissue of Elschnig is supplied exclusively by the ciliary circulation and unfortunately does not receive any contribution from the CRA (Figure 4). There probably would been no chronic glaucoma had the BT received contribution from the CRA as well.

Ciliary circulation is a low-pressure system due to its multiple branches compared to that of the central retinal artery which remains solitary from its origin to its emergence at the ONH. The ciliary systemic perfusion pressure supplying the BT and IOP are opposing forces. Systemic perfusion pressure supplying the BT is normally higher (around 25 mmHg) than the normal range IOP level (10 to 21mmHg) for proper perfusion and healthy maintenance of the BT (Figure 9).

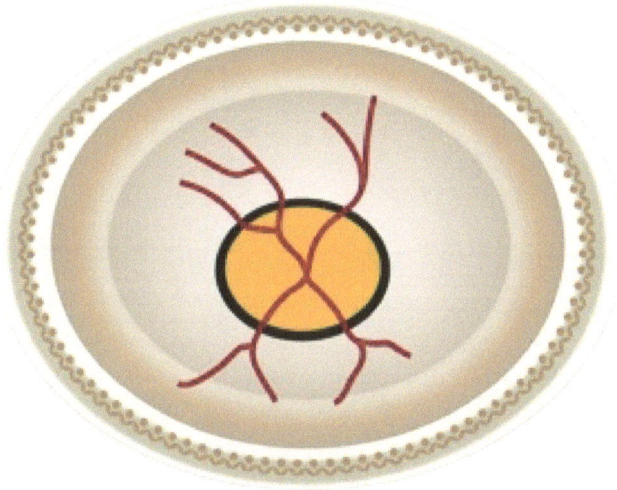

Figure 8. Schematic Diagram. Border tissue of Elschnig (green) keeps the lamina cribrosa firmly in place in the scleral opening. The border tissue appears to be the primary site of injury in glaucoma.

RELATIONSHIP BETWEEN CILIARY PRESSURE AND IOP

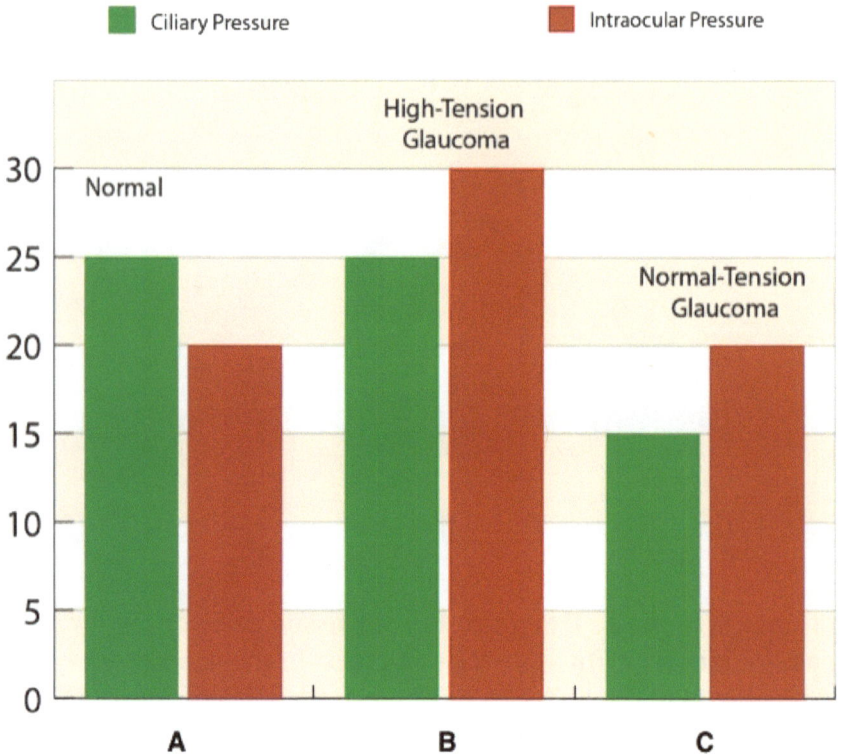

Figure 9. Graphic Diagram. The interaction between ciliary pressure and IOP. Normally, the ciliary pressure supplying the border tissue should be higher than IOP for its good perfusion and healthy maintenance as in column (A). In column (B) the IOP is increased to 30 mmHg due to an ocular problem whereas the ciliary pressure is still the same at 25, resulting in high-tension glaucoma. In column (C), due to decrease of the ciliary pressure to 15 resulting from systemic problems such as hypotension, the normal IOP at 20 mmHg is now acting as an elevated IOP, resulting in normal-tension glaucoma.
Note: In (B) and (C) the situation is reversed - IOP becomes higher than the ciliary pressure. HTG appears to be an ocular problem whereas NTG as a systemic problem.

However, if this healthy relationship is reversed either due to a rise in IOP (e.g. due to an ocular problem) or if the perfusion pressure supplying the BT becomes lower than the IOP due to systemic problems (e.g. chronic hypotension), then even normal IOP will take the upper hand and act as elevated IOP for that subject (Figure 9).

In both scenarios, IOP will act as elevated IOP and chronically compress the ciliary circulation of the BT, resulting in chronic ischemia and its degeneration. Due to degeneration of the BT, the LC will detach from the scleral wall and start sinking in the scleral canal. This will lead to the second, mechanical stage of glaucoma. Thus, it is intraocular pressure whether above the normal level (over 21 mmHg) or within the normal IOP (below 21 mmHg) acting as elevated IOP, being the main cause of glaucoma.

Moreover, chronic glaucoma is indeed a chronic disease as it may take years leading to the degeneration of the BT. A simple analogy: an obese person will require a long period of slow starvation to become emaciated. Total acute starvation would lead to immediate death and there would be no time for emaciation. This compares to acute glaucoma, in which the IOP suddenly becomes extremely elevated and becomes higher than the CRA pressure (around 60 mmHg) and causes acute retinal ischemia and immediate death of the retinal cells.

In acute glaucoma, the IOP becomes higher than CRA pressure which results in acute ischemia of the retina and sudden blindness. However, in chronic glaucoma, the IOP becoming higher than ciliary pressure of the BT, even moderately elevated IOP, will result in chronic ischemia and degeneration of the BT. In other words, IOP is the cause of glaucoma through ischemia in both acute and chronic glaucoma but the mechanisms are different.

In acute glaucoma, the extremely elevated IOP is destroying the NFs by acute ischemia whereas in chronic glaucoma, moderately elevated IOP is causing chronic ischemia of the border tissue leading to its degeneration. Thus resulting in sinking of the LC and leading to severance of NFs.

In both HTG and NTG, IOP is the primary risk factor but there are several secondary factors involved as well in the patho-genesis of glaucoma. In addition to the role of reduced ciliary pressure, the conditions affecting oxygen saturation of the BT such as sleep apnea and smoking will also be contribu-tory factors for degeneration of the BT.

Furthermore, the inherent structural integrity of the BT will be an important factor as well. For example, the thinner BT as in high myopia subjects will lead to its early degeneration. Therefore, chronic glaucoma indeed becomes a multi-factorial disease but IOP is still the only primary risk factor.

It would take longer for degeneration of the BT to occur in subjects with fewer risk factors compared to those with more risk factors. Subjects with fewer risk factors will be able to tolerate elevated IOP for a longer time compared to those with more risk factors. Therefore, their latent pre-perimetric period will be longer. This latent period would vary with each subject. The more risk factors present, the greater the likelihood of rapid degeneration of the BT and thus early development of glaucoma.

The Second Stage: Sinking of the LC and Severance of NFs

The lamina cribrosa (LC), a multilayered rigid connective tissue plate, densely packed with NFs is firmly kept in place in the scleral opening by the border tissue of Elschnig (BT). This border tissue is a collagenous tissue acting as an 'O' ring seal for the lamina cribrosa. In addition to the BT, the 360 degrees of retinal NFs also keeps the LC in place as roots anchor a tree.

Due to degeneration of the border tissue, the LC becomes detached and loose and starts sinking in the scleral canal. As a result, the most peripheral NFs being closest to the scleral edge are stretched and severed first (Figure 10). Thereafter, the next-in-line fiber will move peripherally to the scleral edge to occupy the space vacated by the preceding severed nerve fiber. This next-in-line fiber will then also become severed at the scleral edge.

The severance of NFs leads to further sinking of the LC due to the loss of anchorage provided by the NFs as roots provide anchorage to a tree. This cascade of severance of NFs and sinking of the LC then becomes self-propagated and continues until all the NFs have moved in an orderly tandem fashion to the scleral edge and become severed. The sinking of the LC can explain the orderly destruction of NFs in glaucoma.

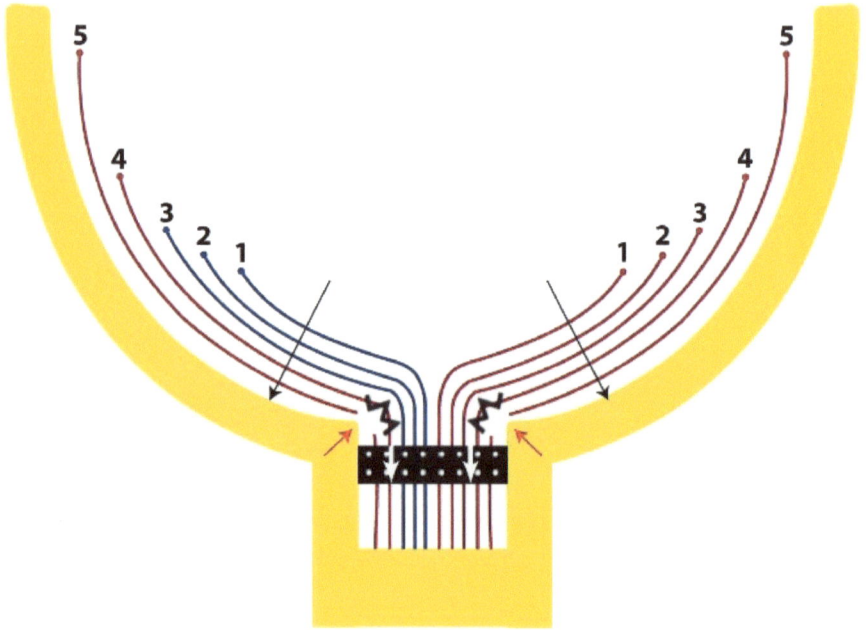

Figure 10. Schematic Diagram. Due to sinking of the LC, the most peripheral and deepest prelaminar nerve fiber (5) was stretched and severed against the scleral edge first (red arrow). The next-in-line fiber (4) will move towards the scleral edge to occupy the space vacated by the preceding severed fiber will also get stretched and severed. This process will continue in an orderly sequence until the most central fiber (1) has moved towards the scleral edge and gets severed (black arrow).

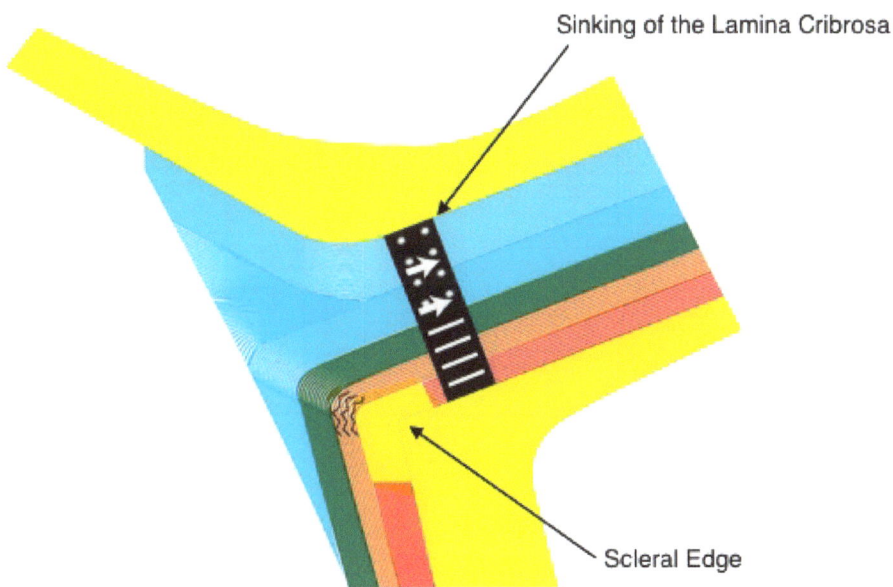

Figure 11. Schematic Diagram. Due to sinking of the LC, the deepest NFs (peripheral vision) being closest to the scleral edge (red) are stretched and severed first. The next-in-line (orange) fibers would move towards the scleral edge and also get stretched and severed. Superficial NFs (central vision) arising closest to the disc (blue) will be the last ones to get severed, maintaining central vision until the end-stage of glaucoma.

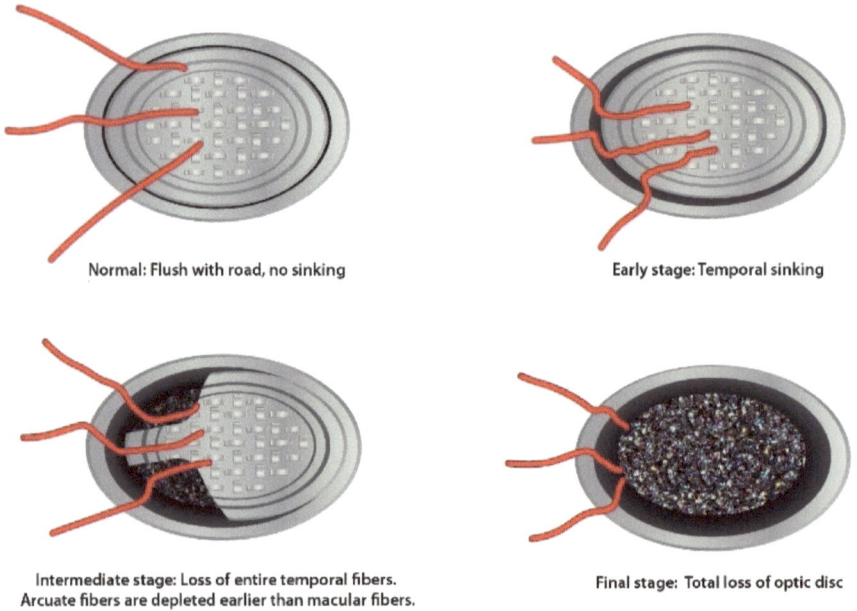

ANALOGY: Manhole Cover to a Glaucomatous Disc

Normal: Flush with road, no sinking

Early stage: Temporal sinking

Intermediate stage: Loss of entire temporal fibers.
Arcuate fibers are depleted earlier than macular fibers.

Final stage: Total loss of optic disc

Figure 12. Schematic Diagram. Analogy of a sinking manhole cover to a glaucomatous disc. The optic disc/LC is sinking usually more temporally, resulting in sloping, kinking of vessels and severance of nerve fibers and vasculature. At the end-stage, all the NFs are severed and optic disc is destroyed - leaving an empty crater.

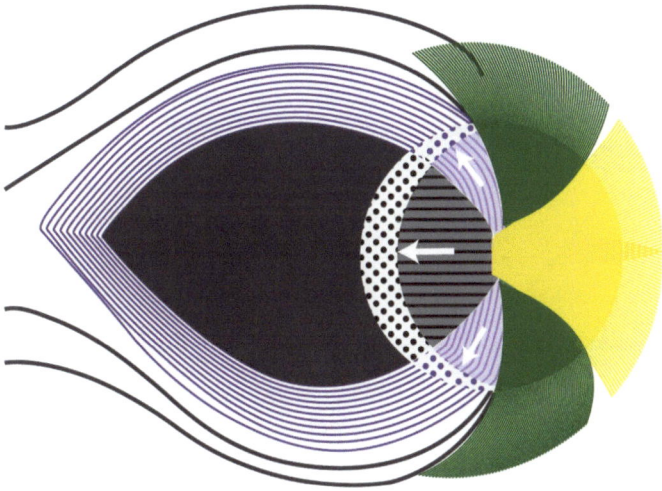

Figure 13. Schematic Diagram. Due to sinking of LC, all the temporal NFs - macular, superior and inferior arcuate - are being severed simultaneously. However, arcuate NFs being fewer in number compared to the macular NFs are depleted earlier, resulting in sharply defined arcuate field defects.

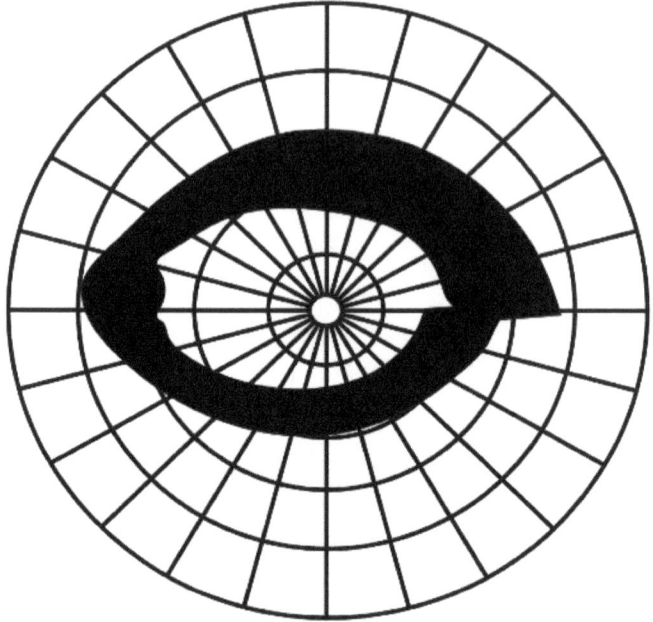

Double arcuate field defect (ring scotoma) in glaucoma

Figure 14. Schematic Diagram. Sharply defined superior and inferior arcuate field defects with nasal step are salient features of glaucoma. Sharply defined margins can only be produced by the selection depletion of the arcuate NFs, not by their atrophy.

The vasculature is also being severed along with the nerve fibers. In essence, the severance of NFs and vasculature is the unique feature of glaucoma as no other disease would cause them.

Do we have evidence of the sinking LC?

The sinking of the LC has been well documented in several published studies. It has been documented that there is posterior migration of the LC from the very early stages of glaucoma thereby substantiating the fact that the optic disc may be sinking in the scleral canal (Young et al, 2011). On the contrary, there is no OCT or histological evidence to prove posterior bowing of the lamina cribrosa or the phenomenon of cupping even though it is commonly believed.

Do we have evidence of severance of nerve fibers and vasculature?

It may not be possible to witness the actual process of severance of NFs. However, we can determine the phenomenon of severance by indirect observation and deductive reasoning.

Progressive thinning of the retinal nerve fiber layer (RNFL) observed through optical coherence tomography (OCT) is the salient feature of glaucoma. The progressive thinning of the RNFL continues until it hits the 'floor effect'. The floor effect is the stage after which we can't measure any further thinning of the RNFL. This floor effect appears to be due to the fact that all the NFs have been severed and that there is nothing left to measure further thinning of the RNFL.

The production of notching (empty spaces) at the superior and inferior poles of the glaucomatous disc is due to depletion of arcuate nerve fibers after their severance. The entire temporal fibers (macular, superior and inferior arcuate) are being severed simultaneously. However, the arcuate fibers being fewer in number compared to the macular fibers are depleted earlier producing arcuate field defects. And notching in the superior and inferior poles of the disc at the site of their entry and wedge shaped empty loss in the retina (Figure 13).

Notching and wedge shaped retinal spaces can only be produced due to severance and depletion of the arcuate NFs. If the NFs were being atrophied, then we wouldn't be seeing notching or empty retinal spaces since the atrophied NFs become shrunken but don't become depleted.

Due to sinking of the LC, the microvasculature is meeting the same fate at the scleral edge as the NFs. Blood capillaries are also being stretched and broken, resulting in splinter hemorrhages at the disc margin and characteristic whitish pallor of the ONH.

OCT angiography (OCTA) has shown the reduced vascular network in glaucoma subjects even in the pre-perimetric stages. Retinal vessel measurements in each area show a stepwise decrease in normal to pre-perimetric and end-stage glaucoma discs.

The reduced vascular density in glaucoma subjects appears to be due to severance of the vasculature. The area around the disc becomes scant of smaller vessels due to their severance and appears bald - a valuable sign in glaucoma.

The nasal shifting of the central vessels in the glaucomatous disc occurs in temporally tilted discs. Although the entire 360 degrees of NFs are being severed, due to the temporal tilt of the optic disc, the temporal NFs are being severed more than the nasal fibers. Thus, the nasal fibers being more in number will pull the central vessels nasally.

A simple analogy to illustrate this is that if roots of a tree are cut more on one side, the tree will move to the opposite side. However, in a flatly inserted optic disc, the 360 degrees of the NFs will be severed equally. Thus, there would be no nasal shifting of the central vessels (Figure 15, 16)

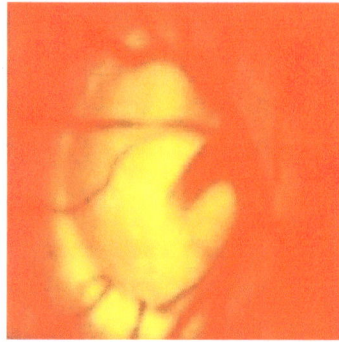

Figure 15. End-stage glaucomatous disc with nasal shifting of central vessels due to unequal severance of NFs - more temporal than nasal in a temporally tilted disc.

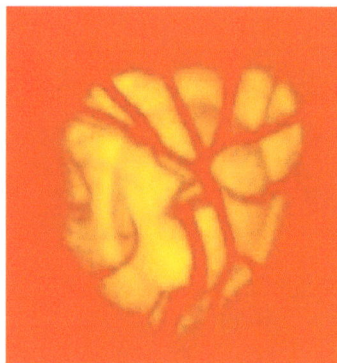

Figure 16. End-stage glaucomatous disc, no nasal shifting of central vessels due to equal 360 degrees severance of NFs in a flatly inserted disc.

The histology of the end-stage glaucomatous disc resembles an empty crater. There are no NFs or blood vessels except for some larger blood vessels still hanging on the scleral edge. The empty crater can only result from severance of NFs and vasculature. In contrast, the end-stage histology of non-glaucomatous optic atrophy such as due to multiple sclerosis reveals presence of NFs though shrunken and disorganized (Figure 17).

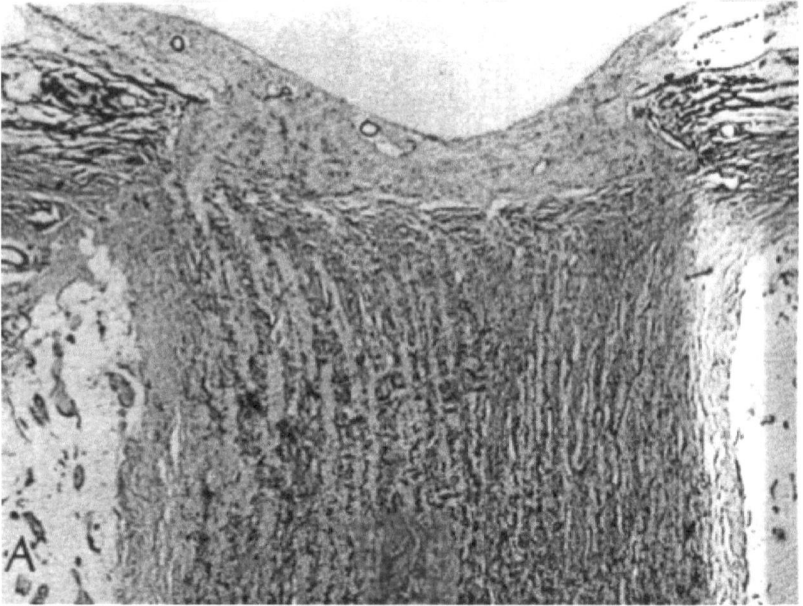

Figure 17. Histology: optic atrophy due to multiple sclerosis.
Note the nerve fibers though shrunken and disorganized are
still present in contrast to total disappearance of NFs in the
end-stage glaucomatous disc (Fig. 18). There is no severance
of NFs and thus no excavation in a non-glaucomatous optic
atrophy. (Image by permission: Yanoff, Ocular Pathology,
Harper & Row, 1975).

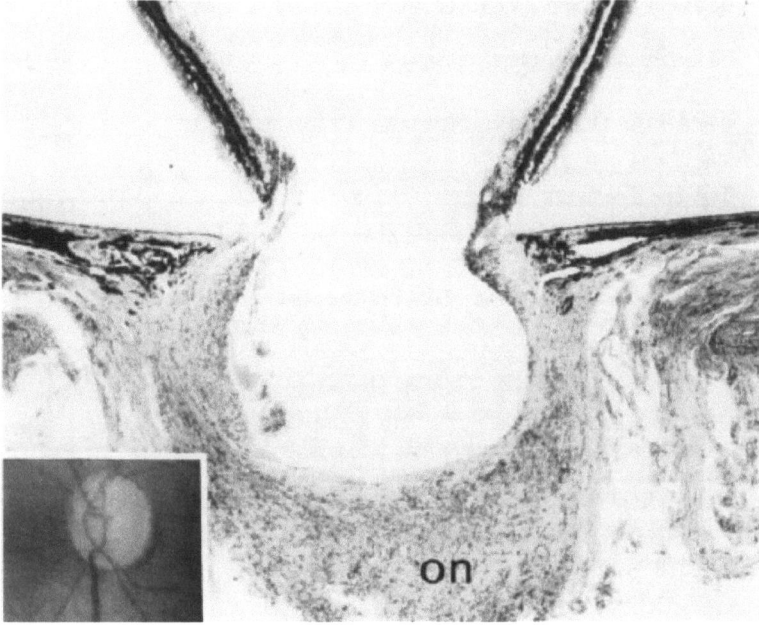

Figure 18. Histology end-stage glaucomatous disc. A large crater left over after severance of nerve fibers. Mistakenly described as 100% cupped LC. (Image by permission: Yanoff, Ocular Pathology, Harper & Row, 1975).

Chapter 6

The Production of Glaucomatous Field Defects

The most pathognomonic feature of glaucomatous field defects is that they are produced in a predictable and orderly sequence. The glaucomatous field defects never occur randomly. If the visual field defects were erratic and unpredictable, we wouldn't be doing perimetry in glaucoma.

In glaucoma, the peripheral visual fields are lost first but they have poor diagnostic value due to normal variation in the extent of the peripheral field. Moreover, diseases like cataracts can also limit the peripheral fields. The production of isolated scotomas in the paracentral region (10 to 20 degrees) are the early diagnostic signs of glaucoma. These isolated scotomas become enlarged and more frequent. They ultimately coalesce to become complete superior and inferior arcuate scotomas which are diagnostic of glaucoma. No other disease creates such a result in this classical way.

The arcuate field defects produced in the early stages of glaucoma, due to destruction of the arcuate nerve fibers, are a pathognomonic feature of both high-tension and normal-tension glaucoma. Although these arcuate field defects were discovered more than 100 years ago by Bjerrum and Ronnie, we still don't have consensus as to why arcuate scotomas are produced.

There are two main theories about the pathogenesis of arcuate field defects: mechanical and vascular. According to the mechanical theory, the superior-temporal and inferior-temporal areas of the LC, containing arcuate fibers, have larger sized pores which are easily compressed by distortion of the LC by elevated IOP. This in turn causes impediment of the axoplasmic flow resulting in the death of RGCs (Quigley, 1981).

The vascular theory suggests that elevated IOP compresses the blood vessels resulting in ischemia and death of the RGCs. Duke-Elder, Henkind, and Harrington were proponents of the vascular theory. Henkind (1967) suggested the occlusion of the radial peripapillary capillaries as the cause of selective destruction of the arcuate fibers. However, some believe that arcuate fibers are destroyed early in glaucoma because they are more sensitive to IOP.

There was a very comprehensive discussion in the "Pathogenesis of Visual Field in Glaucoma" by Edward Maumenee, published in Controversy in Ophthalmology (1977). Maumenee had challenged the direct role of both mechanical and vascular theory for the production of the glaucomatous field defects. Further, he argued against the vascular theory because of normal electroretinogram and fluorescein angiography in glaucoma, which he expected to be abnormal if vascular theory was valid.

He remarked that both mechanical and vascular theories were not convincing and concluded that the exact cause of loss of visual field in glaucoma is not known at present time. This was said in the mid-1970s. Today, we still have no agreement as to the causation of the arcuate field defects.

Although the selective destruction of arcuate nerve fibers is an important feature in early glaucoma, the most distinctive feature is the orderly and systematic loss of NFs, starting with peripheral and ending with the central NFs. The production of arcuate field defects is only a part of the systematic loss of NFs in glaucoma. Both mechanical and ischemic injuries, acting directly on the NFs, can never result in the orderly loss of NFs in glaucoma. Therefore, there should be an indirect way for the orderly destruction of NFs in glaucoma.

Can the sinking LC and severance of NFs corroborate with the orderly loss of glaucomatous field defects?

Likely. The sinking of the LC will lead to stretching and severance of NFs in an orderly sequence from peripheral to central. Due to degeneration of the BT, the LC becomes loose and starts sinking in the scleral canal. As the LC sinks, the most peripheral fibers being closest to the scleral edge would get stretched as one end is attached to the soma of the RGC and the other end is secured in the pores of the LC, and ultimately become severed. This can explain the loss of peripheral visual fields in the early stages of glaucoma.

However, the loss of peripheral fields has little diagnostic value because of normal variation of the limits of the peripheral field. The most diagnostic feature of glaucoma is the production of isolated scotomas in the paracentral area (10 to 20 degrees). The arcuate fibers are also arranged in layers from superficial (closer to vitreous) to deep as the rest of the nerve fibers. Thus, as the LC sinks, the deepest arcuate fibers (closest to sclera) are stretched and severed first resulting in isolated scotomas.

The production of only a few isolated scotomas in the early stages suggest that very few NFs are destroyed first in glaucoma. As more of the arcuate NFs are severed, the scotomas become more frequent and enlarged and ultimately coalesce to become complete superior and inferior arcuate scotomas. When all of the superior and inferior arcuate NFs are severed and depleted, a ring scotoma is produced in the paracentral area (10 to 20 degrees).

Why are the arcuate fibers being selectively destroyed?

As the LC sinks, the entire temporal fibers (macular, superior and inferior arcuate) are being severed simultaneously. However, arcuate fibers being fewer in number compared to the macular fibers, are depleted earlier giving rise to the sharply defined arcuate field defects. The macular fibers last until the end-stage due to their abundance.

Despite current glaucoma theories, these arcuate fibers are not being destroyed due to their undue sensitivity to IOP, increased vulnerability due to their location, or due to their unique blood supply. Lastly, the arcuate fibers are not being destroyed selectively, but being depleted early in glaucoma due to their being fewer in number. It would be inconceivable that atrophy of the NFs occur selectively to the arcuate nerve fibers only in the early stages of glaucoma and not involving the rest of the NFs.

The decrease in thickness of the macular ganglion cell complex observed in the early stages of glaucoma substantiate the fact that macular fibers are also being severed along with rest of the NFs from day one. Arcuate field defects have sharply defined margins which can't be produced if the NFs were being atrophied. The sharply defined margins of the arcuate field defects can only be produced by severance and depletion of NFs, not due to their atrophy.

The nerve fibers in the prelaminar and the laminar region of the ONH are arranged in the way the retinal fibers enter the ONH. After the nerve fibers leave the LC, they are rearranged in temporal and nasal halves inclusive of macular fibers. Since the glaucomatous field defects corroborate with the arrangement of NFs in the prelaminar or laminar region of the ONH, the most likely site of injury in glaucoma is the prelaminar or laminar region of the ONH.

Why are the NFs of the ONH being destroyed one-by-one in an orderly sequence in glaucoma?

The feat of orderly loss of NFs can't be accomplished by any direct ischemic or mechanical insult to the NFs of the ONH due to elevated IOP or otherwise. Moreover, for one-by-one destruction of the NFs, they should be lying loose so they could be easily separated individually. This is only possible when the NFs are lying loose in the prelaminar area and have not yet fastened in bundles in the intricate meshwork of the lamina cribrosa. Once the NFs are fastened in bundles in the LC, their separation into individual nerve fibers is not possible - a prerequisite for the orderly loss of NFs in glaucoma.

In summary, sinking of the LC will result in separation of the prelaminar NFs into individual nerve fibers. The continuous sinking of the LC and severance of NFs will lead to orderly loss of NFs corroborating with glaucomatous field defects. The orderly loss of NFs suggest that the prelaminar area and not the lamina cribrosa can be the site of injury in glaucoma. Moreover, the NFs are being severed, not atrophied in glaucoma. Therefore, glaucoma may not be an optic disc neuropathy, but an optic disc axotomy.

Chapter 7

Risk Factors for Glaucoma

There are primary and secondary risk factors in the pathogenesis of glaucoma.

The Primary Risk Factor: Intraocular Pressure (IOP)

Without doubt, glaucoma is a multi-factorial disease in which several risk factors are playing their role. This occurs when there is elevated IOP (over 21mmHG) or normal IOP acting as elevated IOP. However, IOP is the only primary risk factor for both HTG and NTG. Elevated IOP alone can result in glaucoma without any additional secondary risk factors as evident in traumatic glaucoma.

In the case of unilateral traumatic glaucoma in a healthy subject, moderately elevated IOP is the only risk factor present in the causation of this glaucoma. This presents a puzzling question. If elevated IOP is the cause of glaucoma, then why is normal IOP (less than 21mmHg) causing normal-tension glaucoma?

We have already ruled out the increased sensitivity of the ONH to IOP and other factors in the causation of NTG. I believe that in NTG, IOP even within the normal range, is acting as elevated IOP in that particular subject. As I have hypothesized earlier, the IOP becoming higher than the ciliary pressure of the BT, results in chronic ischemia and degeneration of the border tissue – which is the cause of glaucoma in both HTG and NTG

Once the degeneration of the BT occurs and the LC starts sinking, all chronic glaucomas including NTG behave and follow the same course of disease. This is irrespective of whether elevated IOP was the only risk factor or if it was also facilitated by secondary risk factors as well. We may call glaucoma a multi-factorial disease but ultimately all these factors lead to one final common ground - degeneration of the border tissue, sinking of the LC and severance of NF's.

Secondary Non-IOP Risk Factors

There are three main secondary non-IOP risk factors.

1. Structural integrity of the border tissue

2. Circulatory conditions of the border tissue

3. Oxygenation saturation of the border tissue

1. Structural integrity of the border tissue

The border tissue of Elschnig (BT) is a collagenous tissue which lies between the scleral edge and lamina cribrosa. The BT provides anchorage and keeps the lamina cribrosa in place like an "O" ring seal.

The structural integrity of the BT varies in each individual. Given the same circumstances, the stronger and thicker BT will take a longer time to degenerate compared to a thinner BT. High myopic eyes will have structurally weak and thinner BT due to a bigger scleral opening, while hyperopic eyes will have a smaller scleral opening and thicker and stronger BT.

Thinner and weaker border tissue may be a reason for a higher incidence of glaucoma in cases of high myopia. On the other hand, thicker and stronger border tissue may be the reason for a longer period of pre-perimetric ocular hypertension.

In summary, the inherent strength of the BT is an important factor in the development of glaucoma. Genetics may be playing a role in glaucoma by elevating IOP due to deficient drainage at the trabecular meshwork as in HTG, but genetically structurally weaker border tissue may be playing a role in NTG.

2. Circulatory conditions of the border tissue

Circulatory conditions of the BT are extremely important in the development of glaucoma. The BT is solely supplied by ciliary circulation and it does not receive any contribution from the central retinal artery (CRA). The ciliary circulation supplying the BT is of lower pressure (around 25 mmHG) yet higher than normal range IOP (10 to 21 mmHg). Ciliary circulatory pressure supplying the BT and IOP are opposing forces. Normally, circulatory pressure supplying the BT is higher than IOP for healthy maintenance of the BT.

If either IOP becomes higher than the ciliary pressure due to an ocular problem or the ciliary pressure becomes lower than normal IOP due to systemic problems such as chronic hypotension, then IOP, in both scenarios, will take the upper hand. It will compress the circulation of the border tissue, resulting in chronic ischemia and its degeneration. In the latter scenario, normal IOP becoming higher than ciliary pressure will act as elevated IOP for that subject resulting in NTG. Thus it is IOP, whether elevated or normal (but acting as elevated IOP), which is the culprit in both HTG and NTG (Figure 9).

3. Oxygen saturation of the border tissue

Oxygen saturation of the blood is also important for the healthy maintenance of the BT. Subjects with low oxygen saturation conditions such as sleep apnea, COPD and long - term smokers would be more prone to degeneration of the BT and thus more likely to develop glaucoma.

How do various factors play their role in glaucoma?

The more risk factors present, the more the likelihood of developing glaucoma. For example, if someone has elevated IOP and also has high myopia, chronic hypotension, sleep apnea and long-term smokers will have a much higher risk of early degeneration of BT and rapid progression of glaucoma compared to a subject who has a risk factor of elevated IOP only. The more risk factors present, the earlier the development and severity of glaucoma.

Glaucoma is a complex multi-factorial disease but the bottom line is that all multiple factors lead to one ending - degeneration of the BT which results in LC sinking and severance of NFs. Ocular hypertension is not a benign condition, but is glaucoma in a latent pre-perimetric stage during which the border tissue is undergoing degeneration by chronic ischemia. This latent period will vary in every subject depending upon IOP level and secondary risk factors.

Secondary risk factors are important in the development and progression of glaucoma but most likely none of them can cause glaucoma of its own. They are only piggybacks in subjects with compromised circulation of the BT. I believe secondary risk factors such as high myopia alone can't result in glaucoma in subjects with healthy border tissue circulation. But we should watch for secondary risk factors and prophylactically lower IOP in high risk subjects.

It is mentioned that glaucoma is not a single disease but rather a group of degenerative disorders. I don't agree. I believe chronic glaucoma is a single disease because all cases of chronic glaucoma manifest the same pathological and morphological changes in the disc and produce the same kind of glaucomatous field defects. Without doubt, glaucoma is a multi-factorial disease with a final pathway leading to the sinking of the LC and severance of nerve fibers.

Chapter 8

Questions and Answers

1. Can the lamina cribrosa be the site of injury in glaucoma?

It is widely believed that the lamina cribrosa (LC) is the primary site of injury in glaucoma. It is theorized that elevated IOP causes posterior bowing of the LC (cupping) resulting in distortion of the laminar plates and misalignment of its pores which in turn pinches the axons and thereby impedes the axoplasmic transport leading to death of RGCs. However, it can't be that simple in view of the orderly loss of NFs in glaucoma.

It is inconceivable that the multilayered connective tissue plate, densely packed with NFs, will start bowing posteriorly with an elevation of only 5-10 mmHg of IOP, yet the LC wouldn't bow in cases of acute glaucoma in which the IOP becomes extremely elevated. We never see acute cupping occurring in acute glaucoma.

There is no histology supporting posterior bowing of the LC. Instead, we have evidence of posterior migration of LC, in other words, its detachment from the original insertion from the very early stages of glaucoma, which will itself contradict the posterior bowing of the LC. It is not possible that a loosened and detached LC while migrating posteriorly would also become bowed posteriorly, especially with an elevation of only 5-10 mmHg of IOP.

If the LC was indeed bowing posteriorly, then the central vision fibers should have been destroyed first as they would be located at the apex of the bowed LC. The loss of central vision would have resulted in immediate blindness. But in actuality, the peripheral fibers are being destroyed first while the central vision fibers last until the end-stage of glaucoma.

The intricate meshwork of laminar plates and pores can neither result in the production of sharply defined arcuate field defects nor the orderly loss of NFs in glaucoma. It is incomprehensible that the complex and variable intricate meshwork of the LC pores, densely packed with NFs will always destroy the NFs in an orderly fashion.

Most importantly, for orderly one-by-one loss, the NFs should be loose so they could be easily separated into individual nerve fibers while they are in the prelaminar area. But, once the NFs enter and get fastened in bundles in the pores of the LC, their separation into individual fibers is not possible – a requirement for their orderly loss.

Based on the orderly loss of nerve fibers, the lamina cribrosa cannot be the site of injury in glaucoma.

2. Is glaucoma a neurodegenerative disease?

Glaucoma is theorized as a neurodegenerative disease akin to Alzheimer's, Parkinson's or ALS. In every neurodegenerative disease, the neurons are dying randomly, but in glaucoma the NFs are being destroyed in a specific orderly sequence. This fact alone should keep glaucoma apart from the group of neurodegenerative diseases.

For glaucoma to be a neurodegenerative disease, somehow the RGCs would have to first predict the impending glaucoma so they could start degenerating in an orderly sequence starting with those serving the peripheral vision and ending with those serving the central vision - a very unlikely scenario. I don't believe our RGCs are that smart.

My belief as to why some researchers considered glaucoma to be a neurodegenerative disease is because of the finding of simultaneous death of retinal ganglion cells and of neurons in the lateral geniculate nucleus (LGN) and in the visual cortex.

This occurrence can be explained due to severance of NFs at the scleral edge, resulting in retrograde degeneration of RGCs and anterograde (Wallerian) degeneration of the neurons of the LGN and also of neurons of the visual cortex.

In view of the systematic and orderly loss of NFs, glaucoma couldn't be a neurodegenerative disease.

3. Is glaucoma is due to apoptosis?

It is mentioned that RGCs are undergoing apoptosis (suicide) in glaucoma triggered by elevated IOP. If apoptosis is triggered by elevated IOP, then why is normal IOP triggering normal-tension glaucoma?

Genetically controlled apoptosis is supposed to get rid of randomly occurring old and diseased cells. It is inconceivable that apoptosis in glaucoma will get rid of normal and healthy RGCs especially in an orderly sequence starting with those serving the peripheral vision and ending with RGCs serving the central vision.

If apoptosis is indeed occurring, how can we explain apoptosis in cases of traumatic glaucoma which are not genetically controlled yet the NFs are being destroyed in an orderly sequence. There are other genetic diseases of RGCs such as Tay-Sachs disease which neither result in the orderly loss of NFs nor result in the cupping of the disc.

Based on the orderly loss of NFs, apoptosis has no role in glaucoma.

4. Is glaucoma an optic neuropathy?

Glaucoma is defined as a progressive optic neuropathy. Optic neuropathy is a broad umbrella term which includes both glaucomatous and non-glaucomatous optic atrophies (NGOA). Optic neuropathy of the ONH implies that NFs are being atrophied and shrinking in size. However there are some characteristic morphological and histological changes in the glaucomatous discs which are not occurring in the NGOAs.

The NFs are being destroyed in an orderly and predictable sequence in glaucoma. In contrast, the NFs are being destroyed randomly in the NGOAs. The glaucomatous discs are always excavated whereas NGOAs are non-excavated or flat disc optic atrophies (Figure 27, 28). The histology of end-stage glaucomatous disc reveals an empty crater devoid of NFs whereas the histology of end-stage NGOAs such as due to multiple sclerosis reveals that the NFs are still present, though shrunken and disorganized (Figure 17).

In glaucomatous discs, the blood vessels are sloping and kinking at the disc margin whereas none of these are occurring in NGOAs. In glaucomatous discs, there is usually shifting of the nasal vessels but no such shifting in NGOAs.

The histology of the end-stage glaucomatous disc suggests that NFs are being severed, not atrophied in glaucoma. Therefore glaucoma may not be an optic neuropathy but an optic axotomy.

5. Is normal-tension glaucoma due to non-IOP factors?

Normal-tension glaucoma (NTG) is a glaucoma occurring with IOP consistently within normal levels (10-21 mmHg). In contrast, high-tension glaucoma (HTG) has IOP above the normal level (more than 21 mmHg), which is a statistically selected cut-off number. The bottom line is that though the incidence of glaucoma will increase with increasing elevated IOP, glaucoma also occurs with normal IOP levels as well.

Both HTG and NTG have the same glaucomatous disc changes, visual field defects, and run the same course of disease. This would suggest that the same pathological mechanism is occurring in both HTG and NTG. This mystery needs to be resolved.

Many researchers believe since IOP in NTG is consistently within normal levels, NTG may be due to factors other than intraocular pressure. Many researchers believe that NTG subjects have unduly sensitive optic discs to IOP.

If someone was born with unduly sensitive discs to IOP, then that subject should have developed NTG in early childhood, not after age 50 or more. Therefore, undue sensitivity to IOP does not seem to play any role in NTG.

If NTG is due to increased sensitivity of the ONH to IOP, how can we explain that the optic discs which have survived for decades in the same subjects have suddenly become unduly sensitive to the same level of IOP decades later?

How can we rule out that normal IOP is not the cause of glaucoma? As the name implies, the normal intraocular pressure has a pressure component as well, though statistically normal. Moreover, NTG subjects are responding to pressure lowering eye drops to some extent, so even normal IOP appears to be playing a role in the development of glaucoma.

It is unlikely that NTG is due to undue sensitivity of the ONH to IOP. Normal-tension glaucoma subjects have some associated systemic problems which healthy high-tension glaucoma subjects don't have. High-tension glaucoma subjects are usually healthy and the only risk factor they have is elevated IOP due to an ocular problem.

On the other hand, NTG subjects usually also have cardiovascular or respiratory problems. Cardiovascular problems may include chronic hypotension and vascular dysregulation such as Raynaud's disease. Respiratory problems may include sleep apnea and COPD. We rarely find NTG in healthy subjects except in cases of high myopia. But even in an apparently healthy high myopic subject, there would be some systemic disease, such as being a smoker or exposed to second-hand smoke. I believe high myopia, by itself, can't cause NTG in a healthy subject.

The clinical features of both NTG and HTG are the same. Since high-tension glaucoma is caused by elevated IOP, normal-tension glaucoma must also be caused by normal IOP, however acting as elevated IOP in that particular subject. Some circulatory deficiency appears to have occurred in some component of the ONH that NTGs are developing glaucoma even with normal IOP.

We discussed earlier about the degeneration of border tissue, the relationship between IOP and ciliary pressure supplying the border tissue. Normally the ciliary pressure (around 25 mmHg) is higher than normal IOP (10 to 21mmHg) for the proper perfusion and healthy maintenance of the BT.

However, if this healthy relationship is reversed due to reduced ciliary circulation such as chronic hypotension, so that the ciliary pressure becomes lower than normal IOP, then even normal IOP will act as elevated IOP for that particular subject.

I believe IOP is still the primary cause of glaucoma, even at normal levels, but is acting as elevated IOP thereby resulting in NTG. Thus, IOP becoming higher than the ciliary pressure of the BT is the cause of glaucoma in both HTG and NTG (Figure 9). Non-IOP risk factors are playing only a secondary role in NTG but IOP is the primary risk factor for both HTG and NTG.

6. Is reversal of cupping truly occurring in glaucoma?

It is mentioned that reversal of cupping is occurring when intraocular pressure is drastically lowered by surgical means. I believe it is fallacy. It is an established fact that visual loss in glaucoma is irreversible. Then why should cupping be reversible?

The so-called 'reversal of cupping' has only been observed in cases in which IOP has been drastically reduced by surgery - not when IOP has been lowered by medical treatment. We can't drastically lower the IOP with medical treatment due to a built in safety mechanism. Due to surgery, the built-in safety mechanism gets broken. Therefore the IOP gets lowered too much resulting in hypotony, which in turn results in hyperemia or filling in of the optic cup (Sadun, 1999).

This reduction in the cup size due to hyperemia is mistakenly construed as reversal of cupping. Moreover, this reversal of cupping is only temporary as after a few months it reverses back to the pre-surgical level of cupping which is indicative that reversal of cupping which was originally theorized, was not correct.

Most importantly, if the reversal of cupping was true, then we should have also seen regaining of the vision loss and visual fields defects - which are not occurring. Thus, the reversal of cupping is not genuine and appears to be a misinterpretation.

7. Is the optic disc doughnut shaped?

It is widely mentioned that all NFs of the ONH are present only in the so-called neuroretinal rim while the central cupped area is a hole devoid of NFs – analogous to a doughnut.

There is no histology available supportive of doughnut shaped configuration of the NFs in any ONH normal or diseased. The histology of all of the ONH, glaucomatous or otherwise reveal the LC fully packed with NFs all the way to the center and there is no central empty space or hole except for the central retinal vessels.

The physiological cups are a fibrous tissue remnant of Bergmeister's papilla. The larger the remnant tissue, the larger the size of the cup. In the histology of normal discs, this remnant tissue is identified as the central meniscus of *Kuhnt* lying superficially on the surface of the nerve fiber layer. Underneath this meniscus, the LC is fully packed with NFs all the way to the center of the disc. In other words, there is no hole present (Figure 7).

In fact, the neuroretinal rim is the exposed part of the nerve fiber layer, in other words, the area uncovered by the meniscus. Histology reveals the NFs are present underneath the meniscus as well.

If the ONH was indeed doughnut shaped, then the discs with larger cups or holes should be less likely to develop glaucoma since most of the IOP force will be dissipated in the larger hole and the neuroretinal rim would escape injury. Therefore, the larger the central hole, the less likelihood of neuroretinal rim getting injured contrary to current belief that discs with larger cups are more prone to developing glaucoma.

In a nutshell, the concept of neuroretinal rim and doughnut shaped configuration of the ONH is misinterpreted since there is no histological evidence available to substantiate it.

8. Is glaucoma due to low CSF Pressure?

It is postulated that the lamina cribrosa separates the cerebrospinal fluid and intraocular fluid, both exerting opposing pressure on the LC. Thus, the LC is acting as a fulcrum. Researchers have hypothesized that if CSF pressure is lower than the IOP, the LC will bow posteriorly. Conversely, if CSF pressure is higher than IOP, the LC will bow anteriorly.

The normal CSF pressure is about 8-15 mmHg whereas normal range IOP is 10 to 21 mmHg. Therefore, statistically, at least 50% of subjects should be having CSF pressure lower than IOP. In other words, about 50% of the general population should be developing glaucoma. But glaucoma involves only about 2% of the general population.

It is hard to comprehend that the multilayered rigid LC, densely packed with one million or so NFs is so flimsy that it would move back and forth with just a rise and fall of about 5-10 mmHg of IOP yet it would not bow in cases of acute glaucoma where IOP becomes extremely elevated (70 mmHg or above). If the LC was so flimsy, we should have observed acute cupping occurring in acute glaucomas as well – which is not happening.

The low CSF pressure compared to IOP is theorized to be resulting in posterior bowing of the LC. Nevertheless, we have already rejected the concept of cupping in the context of the orderly loss of NFs in glaucoma.

In view of the aforementioned, CSF pressure has no role in glaucoma.

9. Is thinner cornea a risk factor for glaucoma?

Thinner cornea by itself cannot be a risk factor since glaucoma is a disease of the ONH, not of the cornea. The only exception may be in cases where subjects with thinner cornea may also have thinner border tissue that could be more easily degenerated than normal thickness BT under the same circumstances. Although the thinner cornea may measure IOP readings lower than the actual IOP level, the thinner cornea by itself may not be a risk factor.

10. Is larger vertical cup-to-disc ratio a risk factor for glaucoma?

It is stated that larger vertical cup-to-disc ratio is a risk factor for glaucoma. If the larger vertical cup-to-disc ratio is a risk factor, then the question arises why a larger horizontal cup-to-disc ratio is not a risk factor? Unless we have a reason for larger vertical cup-to-disc ratio being a risk factor for glaucoma, it can't be scientifically acceptable. Vertically or horizontally elongated physiological cups are nothing more than the fibrous tissue remnant of Bergmeister's papilla. Why should a fibrous tissue enlarge in response to elevated IOP? The concept of cup-to-disc ratio is wrongly implicated in glaucoma.

I believe the physiological cups become vertically elongated due to the production of notching at the superior and inferior poles of the disc. Notching (empty spaces) is produced due to severance and depletion of the arcuate nerve fibers at the site of their entry in the disc. Thus, the vertically elongated cup may be an acquired phenomenon and representing cases of early glaucoma rather than being a risk factor for glaucoma.

11. Is ocular perfusion pressure important in glaucoma?

Reduced ocular perfusion pressure (OPP) has been considered a risk factor for glaucoma especially in cases of normal-tension glaucoma. However, the optic disc has a dual blood supply: central retinal artery and ciliary circulation. Researchers usually talk about central retinal artery (CRA) pressure since the OPP is described as central retinal artery pressure minus IOP. Ironically, we don't talk about the OPP of the ciliary circulation.

It is observed that OPP is lower in NTG subjects. The question arises as to how is the reduced OPP of CRA causing the orderly loss of NFs in glaucoma? Unless we have the answer, postulating reduced OPP as a cause of NTG is just not enough.

My belief is that OPP of the central retinal artery has no role in the pathogenesis of chronic glaucoma but is involved in acute glaucoma. The CRA has a much higher pressure (around 60 mmHg) than the normal IOP (10 to 21 mmHg) so the retinal circulation remains unimpeded until IOP reaches around 60 mmHg or above. Therefore, when the IOP is elevated above 60 mmHg, as in acute glaucoma, the retinal circulation will be compressed and compromised leading to acute ischemia and the sudden death of the entire retina and no orderly loss of NFs in acute glaucoma.

However, the situation is different in chronic glaucoma as the IOPs are only moderately elevated or even in normal range. Chronic glaucoma can occur with only a 10-15 mmHg elevation of IOP but this elevation has to be on a long-term chronic basis. This suggests that CRA circulation plays a role in acute glaucoma but not in chronic glaucoma. If impairment of CRA circulation can't result in the orderly loss of NF's, then it has no role in the causation of chronic glaucoma. We are then left with the ciliary circulation.

I propose that it is the IOP becoming higher than the perfusion pressure of the border tissue (ciliary circulation) resulting in chronic ischemia and its degeneration; the cause of both HTG and NTG as we have already discussed in this book. In chronic glaucoma, we should be measuring the OPP of ciliary circulation and not of the central retinal artery.

12. Why can't we stop glaucoma despite maximal lowering of IOP?

I have hypothesized that glaucoma is a two-stage disease, biological and mechanical. The LC is anchored in the scleral opening by the border tissue, and also by the 360 degrees of retinal NFs as roots anchor a tree. As the LC sinks in the scleral canal, the NFs are stretched and severed at the scleral edge. The severance of additional NFs leads to further LC sinking due to loss of anchorage provided by the NFs.

The cascade of severance of NFs and sinking of LC would self-propagate and continue until all the NFs have moved in an orderly tandem sequence to the scleral edge and become severed (Figure 10). This may explain the unstoppable nature of glaucoma despite maximum lowering of IOP. We may be slowing the progression of glaucoma by lowering IOP but can't halt it completely due to the mechanical nature of the disease.

13. Do cup-to-disc ratios have any validity in glaucoma diagnosis?

Physiological cups are fibrous tissue remnants of Bergmeister's papilla, identified in the histology as the central meniscus of *Kuhnt* lying superficially on the nerve fiber layer. Underneath this meniscus, the LC is densely packed with NFs all the way to the center (Figure 7). The fibrous tissue base of physiological cups is not enlarging but breaking up in glaucoma due to sinking and severance of NFs. Therefore, cup-to-disc ratios have no validity in glaucoma. They are misleading in glaucoma diagnosis.

14. Is ocular hypertension a benign disease?

Ocular hypertension is the pre-perimetric and latent stage of glaucoma in which degeneration of the border tissue is taking place. The latent period varies in subjects depending upon the severity of IOP and multiplicity of the secondary risk factors as we have already discussed. Ocular hypertension is not a benign disease. It is a pre-perimetric glaucoma and should be treated. Sooner or later ocular hypertension will manifest into glaucoma.

15. Is the end-stage glaucomatous disc a 100% cupped lamina cribrosa?

It is widely described that the end-stage glaucomatous disc is a 100% cupped lamina cribrosa - also described as an empty bean-pot. There are two important issues regarding histology of the end-stage glaucomatous disc.

First, it is inconceivable that the multilayered rigid LC is so stretchable that it would become cupped or ballooned in the shape of a large empty bean-pot. Second, why is the bean-pot empty? Where did the nerve fibers and its vasculature go?

The histology of the end-stage non-glaucomatous optic disc atrophy such as due to multiple sclerosis reveals the presence of NFs, though shrunken and disorganized (Figure 17). However, there are no NFs present in the end-stage glaucomatous disc (Figure 18).

The absence of NFs and vasculature in the end-stage glaucomatous disc can only be explained by their severance and subsequent phagocytosis. If we look closely at histology of the end-stage glaucomatous disc, we will find that it is not a 100% cupped LC but a crater left over after the severance of nerve fibers. The histology of the end-stage glaucoma disc speaks for itself - glaucoma may not be an optic neuropathy but an optic axotomy.

Chapter 9

A Simple Method to Diagnose Glaucoma

In medicine, we diagnose a disease based on the pathological changes pertinent and unique to that disease. However, we are diagnosing glaucoma based on cupping which may not be occurring at all. As a result, there is wide variation in glaucoma diagnosis even among experts because we are looking at changes in the glaucomatous disc which are not pertinent to this disease.

A simple method to diagnose glaucoma is based on the sinking disc/LC, severance of NFs and vasculature, which I believe are occurring in the glaucomatous disc. In order to examine the optic disc under this method, we will have to ignore the physiological cups whether they have a cup-to-disc ratio of 0.2 or 0.9. Physiological cups are fibrous tissue remnants of Bergmeister's papilla and have nothing to do with glaucoma. We will have to abandon the terms cupping and cup-to-disc ratio. The term cupping is misleading and we should not be using it in glaucoma. Moreover, we are using the term cupping in describing the physiological cups. By using this term in describing glaucomatous discs, we are creating unnecessary confusion.

It is a fallacy that physiological cups are enlarging concentrically in glaucoma. Why should a fibrous tissue remnant enlarge at all due to elevated IOP especially concentrically thereby defying the laws of physics?

Physiological cups are not enlarging but breaking starting with the production of notching or localized excavation (empty spaces) at the superior and inferior poles and ending with total excavation of the ONH due to severance of NFs in glaucoma.

There are three main events simultaneously occurring in the glaucomatous disc. First, the optic disc/LC is sinking. Second, the NFs are being severed. Third, capillaries and smaller vasculature are also being severed. We will have to take into account all these scenarios while evaluating the glaucomatous disc.

First, normally the blood vessels crossing the disc margin are straight as the optic disc is flushed with the retina. As the optic disc starts sinking, the blood vessels start sloping on the surface of the disc in pursuit of the sinking LC. This is more noticeable in the temporal part of the disc. Sloping of the vessels would be indicative of the sinking disc. If there is no sinking disc, there should be no glaucoma.

Second, due to sinking of the LC, the NFs get stretched and severed. The severance of NFs will produce empty spaces or excavation. The first sign of excavation will be the production of notching at the poles of the disc due to severance and depletion of arcuate fibers – at the site of their entry in the disc. Once notching becomes evident, glaucoma diagnosis is confirmed.

Third, as the LC sinks, the microvasculature and capillaries at the disc margin are also being stretched and broken - meeting the same fate as that of nerve fibers at the scleral edge. The severance of the microvasculature will produce temporal pallor and splinter hemorrhages at the disc margin. Pallor of the optic disc, usually in the temporal region, is the earliest sign of glaucoma prior to sloping of vessels and notching at the poles.

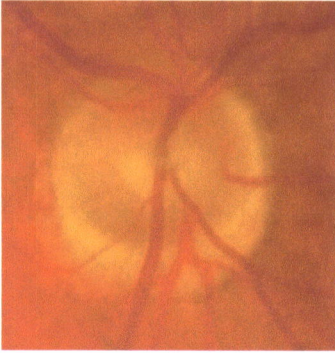
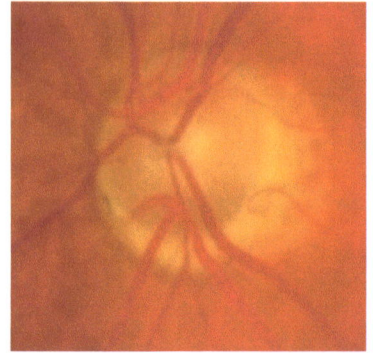

Figure 19. Glaucomatous disc same patient. Uniform sinking of disc in both eyes. Sloping of vessels, no change in the contour of physiological cups. Prominent scleral edge due to thinning of the RNFL.

If the entire 360 degrees of the optic disc is of uniform reddish color and has no pallor, especially in the temporal area, then there should be no glaucoma. As the glaucoma progresses and more of the NFs are severed, more excavation will be produced. Excavation will appear as a depression due to loss of NFs.

It is the excavation or empty spaces which are occurring in the glaucomatous disc, which we misinterpret as cupping. As more of the vasculature is severed, the characteristic whitish pallor will become more pronounced. The depressed and excavated, whitish pale disc along with nasal shifting of the central vessels is characteristic of the glaucomatous disc.

Why are the central vessels shifting nasally?

The nasal shifting of the central vessels is occurring due to severance of NFs. Nasal shifting of the vessels occurs in the temporally tilted optic discs which are more common than flatly inserted discs. Although the entire 360 degrees of NFs are being severed simultaneously, the temporal fibers are being severed more than nasal fibers due to the temporal tilt of the disc. The nasal fibers being more in number than the temporal fibers will pull the central vessels towards its own side (nasally).

An analogy: if more roots of a tree are cut on one side, the tree will shift to the opposite side. In the flatly placed optic disc, nasal shifting of central vessels may not occur since the entire 360 degrees of NFs are being severed equally (Figure 15, 16).

We have to keep in mind that glaucoma is a progressive and unstoppable disease. The LC is anchored in the scleral canal as roots anchor a tree. As the NFs are being severed, the LC sinks further due to loss of anchorage and results in severance of additional NFs. This cascade of the sinking LC and severance of NFs will become self-propagated and will continue until all the nerve fibers are severed and depleted.

The sinking of the LC and severance of NFs along with vasculature are occurring simultaneously. Sinking, excavation and the characteristic whitish pallor gradually become more pronounced as the glaucoma progresses.

We will apply the aforementioned features in the evaluation of the glaucomatous disc. Although the changes occurring in the glaucomatous discs are gradual and continuous, we have arbitrarily divided the glaucomatous disc into three stages.

EARLY STAGE

Although the entire 360 degrees of NFs are being severed simultaneously, the temporal fibers are being severed more than nasal fibers due to the inherent temporal tilt. The temporal area will appear pale due to severance of the microvasculature in the early stages. Pallor of the disc will become obvious sooner than the sloping of the vessels and sinking of the disc.

The temporal scleral edge will appear prominent and visible due to thinning of the RNFL resulting from their severance. In other words, the underlying structures are becoming more visible due to shaving or thinning of the nerve fiber layer. Increased visibility of the scleral edge will be indicative of thinning of the RNFL.

Splinter hemorrhages may also begin to appear at the disc margin due to severance of the blood capillaries. Temporal pallor and splinter hemorrhages will be noticeable prior to any change in the contour of the physiological cup.

As the sinking of the LC progresses and the RNFL thins further, the scleral edge will become even more visible and the temporal blood vessels will appear to begin sloping on the disc surface.

In summary, in the early stages of glaucoma, the temporal area will appear depressed and shallow due to a combination of sinking of LC and diminution of NFs. The temporal scleral edge will appear more visible due to thinning of the RNFL.

The temporal area will appear pale and blanched due to severance of microvasculature – a very important sign of the early glaucomatous disc. If there is no temporal pallor, there is no glaucoma.

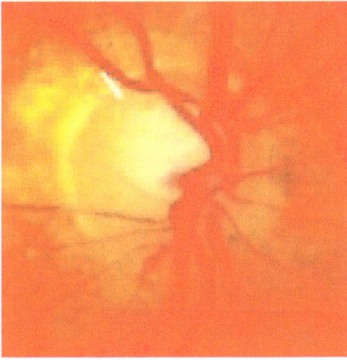 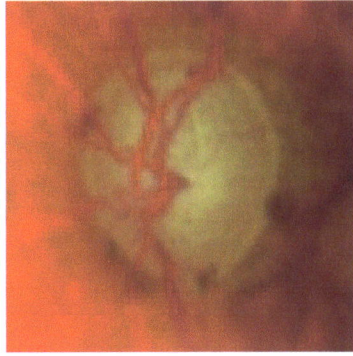

A   B

Figure 20. Glaucomatous disc same patient. A. Early stage right eye: prominent temporal scleral edge due to thinning of RNFL. Temporal pallor and sloping of blood vessels. No change in size of cup. B. Late-stage left eye: excavated disc due severance of NFs. Kinking of blood vessels at the scleral edge due to sinking LC and loss of NFs. Loss of smaller temporal vessels due to their severance. Nasal shifting of central vessels.

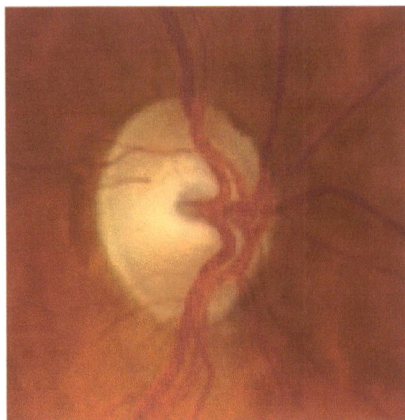 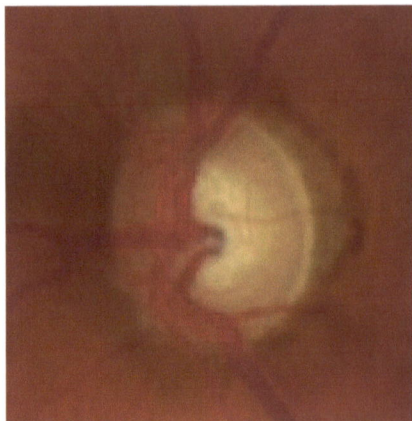

A   B

Figure 21. Glaucomatous disc same patient. A. Early-stage right eye: temporal pallor due to severance of smaller vasculature. No change in size of physiological cup.
B. Later-stage left eye: more temporal pallor. Prominent temporal scleral edge. Cup size still the same.

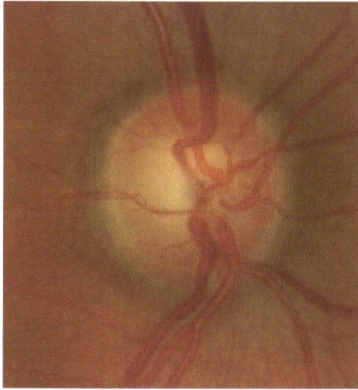 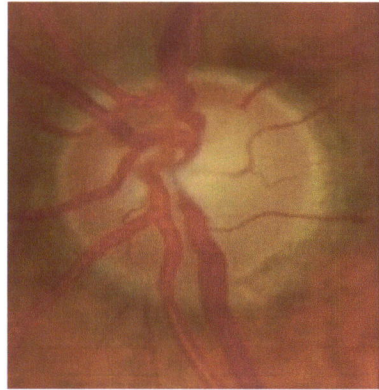

A   B

Figure 22. Glaucomatous disc same Patient. A. Early-stage right eye: temporal pallor and sloping of temporal vessels. Prominent scleral edge due to thinning of RNFL. Cup still intact. B. Later-stage left eye: more obvious uniform sinking of LC, increased sloping of vessels and visibility of 360 degrees of scleral opening.

INTERMEDIATE STAGE

As glaucoma progresses, more of the NFs are severed and depleted. The arcuate fibers, being fewer in number, will be depleted earlier, resulting in production of notching at the superior and inferior poles – the site of their entry in the disc. Notching will be the earliest sign of excavation in glaucoma and will break the physiological cup if present. Physiological cups are not enlarging but breaking up due to production of notching.

When the physiological cup is broken and obliterated, the glaucomatous disc may be called intermediate stage. When notching becomes evident, the arcuate field defects will appear in the paracentral area (10-20 degrees). Notching implies that most if not all of the arcuate NFs have been depleted. At this time, we may observe wedge-shaped retinal defects leading to notching at the poles due to depletion of arcuate NFs.

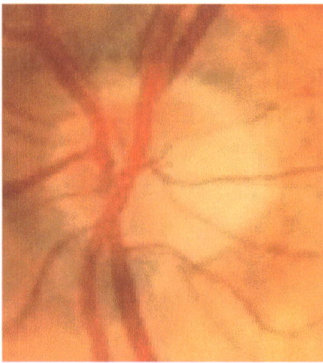
A

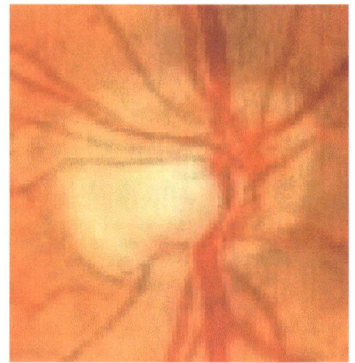
B

Figure 23. Glaucomatous disc same patient. A. Early-stage left eye: temporal pallor and prominent scleral edge due to thinning of RNFL. B. Later-stage right eye: inferior temporal pallor and excavation, sloping of vessels, prominent scleral edge, superior arcuate field defect present.

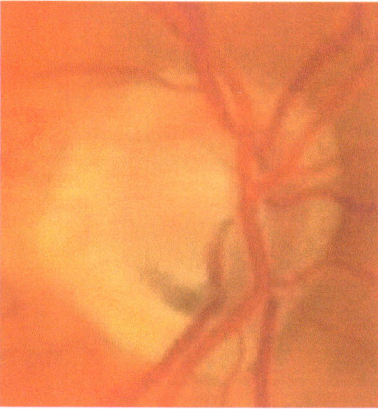

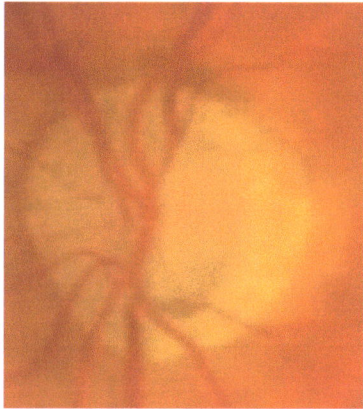

Figure 24. Glaucomatous disc same patient. Uniform sinking in small physiological cup disc in each eye. There is hardly any change in the physiological cup. Sloping of vessels and entire scleral opening becoming more visible due to thinning of RNFL.

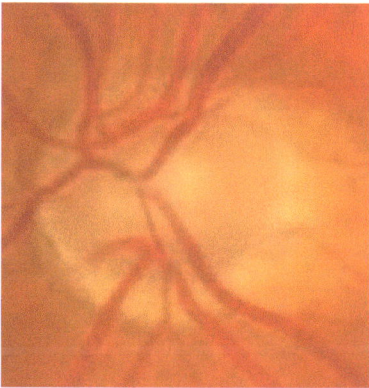

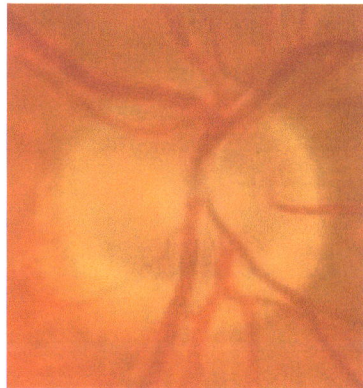

Figure 25. Glaucomatous disc same patient. Uniform sinking in small physiological cup disc in each eye. There is no change in the contour of the physiological cup.

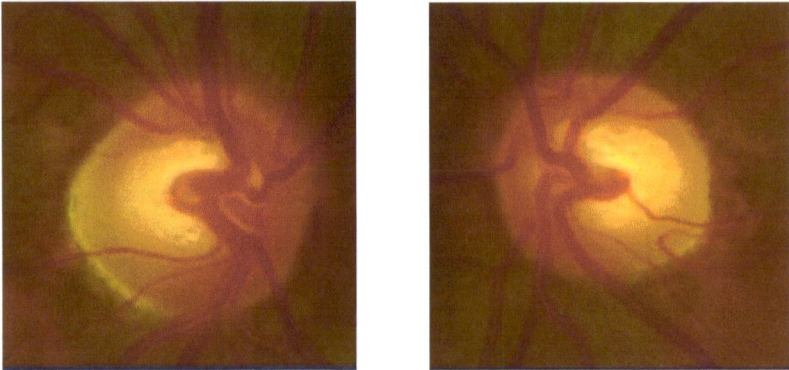

Figure 26. Early glaucomatous disc same patient with Raynaud's disease. Both eyes: temporal pallor, prominent temporal scleral edge, sloping of vessels. Physiological cups still intact and defined. IOP normal. Visual field loss present.

The sloping of the blood vessels will turn into kinking at the site of notching due to severance and loss of underlying NFs. Splinter hemorrhages may be seen at the site of notching due to severance of capillaries since both NFs and micro-vasculature are being severed simultaneously. The underlying scleral edge will become even more visible due to thinning of the RNFL.

As sinking of the LC progresses, the physiological cup will be obliterated due to excavation. At this stage, the physiological cup's usual pallor will become confluent with temporal whitish pallor produced by severance of the vasculature. Blood vessels around the disc will be less in number and the area surrounding the disc will appear bald due to disappearance of smaller blood vessels - a very valuable sign. The central vessels will begin to shift nasally due to loss of anchorage resulting from severance of temporal fibers.

LATE TO END-STAGE

In the late stages of glaucoma, the optic disc surface will be more depressed and excavated due to loss of NFs. Due to extreme thinning of the RNFL, the entire scleral foramen will become more visible. The characteristic whitish pallor will increase greatly due to progressive severance of the vasculature. Smaller blood vessels around the disc will be less in number while those remaining will be kinking at the disc margin due to loss of underlying NFs. In the final stages, there is extreme nasal shifting of central vessels and the rest of the disc area will appear whitish pale and sunken.

The histology of the end-stage glaucomatous disc reveals an empty crater - larger than the size of the original disc, due to loss of neural and glial tissue. There are no visible nerve fibers and vasculature except for some larger blood vessels still hanging over the scleral edge.

In summary, the changes from the early to end-stage glaucomatous disc can be corroborated with gradual sinking of the LC, progressive severance of NFs and of the vasculature. If we keep these events in mind, we would be able to determine any glaucomatous stage easily without reference to cupping or cup-to-disc ratios.

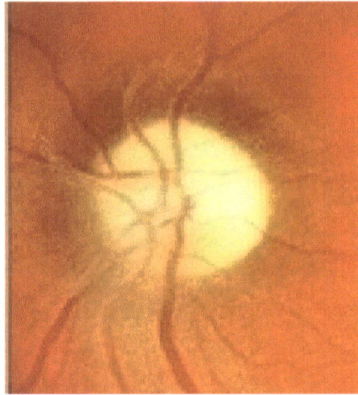

Figure 27. Non- glaucomatous optic atrophy (flat disc atrophy). No sinking of LC. No sloping of vessels. No severance of nerve fibers - no excavation.

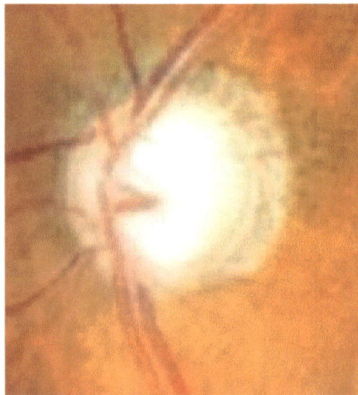

Figure 28. End stage glaucomatous disc: excavated due to severance of NFs. Characteristic whitish pallor due to severance of vasculature. Absence of smaller vessels due to their severance. Nasal shifting of central vessels.

Chapter 10

Treatment of Glaucoma

The intraocular pressure is the primary risk factor for both high-tension (HTG) and normal-tension glaucoma (NTG). If the IOP level is 21 mmHg or higher the glaucoma is called HTG, whereas if IOP is 21mmHg or lower it is called NTG. The normal range of IOP (10 to 21 mmHg) is a statistically selected number by ophthalmologists. The main point is that glaucoma is not only occurring with elevated IOP but also when IOP is consistently within the normal range. It is estimated that that HTG and NTG are about equally distributed in the general population.

During routine eye exam, the measurement of IOP may only be ruling out diagnosis of HTG but not NTG. Therefore, glaucoma screening would not be complete unless it is always accompanied by careful analysis of the ONH in every subject.

Glaucoma is definitively caused either by elevated IOP as in HTG or by normal IOP acting as elevated IOP as in NTG. It is logical to lower the IOP in both HTG and NTG to lower normal levels - around 12 mmHg. By lowering the IOP, we are indirectly improving the profusion of the border tissue of Elschnig.

However, I believe that lowering the IOP below 12 mmHg may not add any further benefit. Furthermore, it may be extremely difficult to lower IOP below 12 mmHg by combination of eye drops and oral treatment due to the inherently built-in safety mechanism of the eye, unless surgically reduced.

I believe our aim should be to keep the IOP lower than 15 mmHg which most likely will be the lowest ciliary pressure of the BT in subjects. Drastic lowering of IOP below 10 mmHg by surgical means can be counter productive as we may encounter surgical complications such as hypotony which would be worse than glaucoma itself and may thus precipitate early total blindness.

However, the lowering of IOP alone may not be enough. We also would have to take into account non-IOP risk factors such as COPD, sleep apnea, chronic hypotension and smoking in every glaucoma subject. We will have to work in collaboration with their internists for treatment of these conditions. Also, in cases of hypertension, advise their internists not to lower their blood pressure too much as it would result in lack of perfusion at the ONH.

Ocular hypertension is not a benign condition but a pre-perimetric glaucoma which should be treated. These subjects would be the lucky ones to be caught up in their early glaucoma stages and should not be deprived of treatment. Internists always treat every hypertension subject, so why shouldn't we be treating every ocular hypertension subject?

Since I believe that NFs are being severed in glaucoma, the end-stage glaucomatous disc would have only a few NFs intact akin to a tree standing with only a few roots. Therefore, it may be prudent to avoid cataract/glaucoma surgery in the late stages of glaucoma as the trauma of surgery may accelerate the breakage of the remaining NFs resulting in early total blindness. An analogy to this would be a tree standing with only a few roots falling even with a small amount of wind.

The prophylactic use of IOP lowering

Since chronic glaucoma is primarily caused by elevated IOP or normal IOP acting as elevated IOP, it would be logical to prophylactically lower the IOP in every subject or at least in those with secondary risk factors. Lowering of the IOP is the most effective neuroprotective agent available which should be utilized prophylactically. Internists are using statins and aspirin to lower the risk of cardiovascular disease prophylactically with great success.

Since the second stage of glaucoma is the mechanical scenario due to sinking of the LC, we may find a therapeutic way to stabilize the sinking LC in the future. Until then, lowering of IOP is the best neuroprotective agent at this time.

Chapter 11

Time for a Paradigm Change

Chronic glaucoma is a perplexing disease ever since it was given a separate entity in the 1850s. Despite extensive research, the exact pathogenesis of glaucoma still remains elusive. I believe we are not making progress in glaucoma because we are working under the wrong paradigm of 'cupping' mistakenly given over 160 years ago.

Ironically, we have done extensive research on every aspect of glaucoma, but not on the concept of cupping itself. We have taken for granted that the cupping concept, given over a century ago, is a foregone conclusion. Since no questions were asked about the validity of cupping, the cupping paradigm became more and more firmly embedded with every generation. The prevalent glaucoma theories are in the context of cupping. In this book, I have put forward my arguments against the concept of cupping.

Why are we still following the wrong cupping paradigm?

The answer is complex and may lie in Thomas Kuhn's landmark book, *The Structure of Scientific Revolutions.*

According to Kuhn, a great philosopher of science:

"The scientific community cannot practice its trade without some framework of concepts and theories known as a paradigm. Once a paradigm gets firmly established, it can be declared invalid only if an alternate candidate is available to take its place. To reject one paradigm without simultaneously substituting another is to reject science itself."

In other words, a current paradigm can never be replaced until an alternate paradigm is available to take its place. Kuhn also argues:

"That scientists are so deeply committed to the reality of their paradigms that it is difficult and even painful for them to give it up."

There appears to be some truth in Kuhn's statement. The term cupping was introduced by simple observation of the glaucomatous disc with a newly invented rudimentary ophthalmoscope 160 years ago. Ophthalmologists during that time found that the glaucomatous discs appeared cupped instead of normally being flat. Therefore, the term cupping was given. Since then, the term cupping has become synonymous with glaucoma and persists to this day.

Over the course of time, instead of checking the validity of cupping, we have postulated several glaucoma theories to justify and enforce the concept of cupping. We have introduced the cup-to-disc ratio, considering that the physiological cups start enlarging concentrically in response to elevated IOP, for which we have no histological proof.

We also have theorized that the lamina cribrosa bows posteriorly or in other words becomes cupped in response to elevated IOP for which there is also no histological evidence. Although we have OCT evidence of posterior sliding of the LC from the very early stages of glaucoma, we still call it cupping and don't seem to abandon the cupping paradigm. In other words, we still acknowledge the LC is bowing posteriorly (cupping) in glaucoma despite the fact that it is proven by OCT that the LC instead is sliding posteriorly, from the very early stages of glaucoma.

How could a loosened and detached LC while migrating posteriorly also become bowed posteriorly especially with an elevation of just 10 mmHg of IOP, yet the LC wouldn't bow in acute glaucoma where the IOP becomes extremely elevated to 60 mmHg or more? We don't see any acute cupping occurring in acute glaucoma. Moreover, it is widely believed that the arrangement of NFs in the ONH is an analogue to a doughnut for which we have no histological proof. I believe this misconception is theorized to justify the cupping paradigm.

In his book, Kuhn further argues:

"Scientists are constantly faced with mismatches between observation and theory. This starts from the moment of the theory being created and continues right up until it is abandoned. Therefore, the old story that scientists are so open minded that they are ready to abandon their theories if it doesn't match observation is not true either. On the contrary, a scientist's primary job is to figure out how to fit observation to a theory. So it turns out that apologetics is one of the most important aspects of true science."

We have made a mountain of the term cupping which started with a simple observation 160 years ago. So, what will happen to decades of research if one day we all agree that the term cupping was mistakenly given?

According to Kuhn:

"Almost every significant breakthrough in the field of scientific endeavor is first a break with tradition, with old ways of thinking, with old paradigms."

I believe it is time to have a critical look into the cupping paradigm. We should not take for granted that a 160 year- old cupping paradigm is correct. Even though some ophthalmologists don't agree with the concept of cupping, they fail to openly denounce the cupping paradigm. Such a failure is unfortunate to our patients and to our profession.

The use of cup-to-disc ratio is creating conundrum in glaucoma diagnosis. Subjects including children born with large physiological cups but with normal IOP are being treated as NTG. It is the duty of glaucoma researchers to either prove the phenomenon of cupping or discard it from glaucoma once and for all.

I believe all the morphological and histological evidence of the glaucomatous optic disc is supportive of the sinking disc and severance of NFs. The only thing we need to change: to look at the glaucomatous disc in the context of sinking LC and severance of NFs and its vasculature. By doing this, we will be seeing true changes in the glaucomatous disc which we have never seen before - a Gestalt switch. It will provide us so much genuine information that we may not need anything else.

As once quoted by Albert Szent-Gyorgyi (Nobel Laureate, 1937):

"Discovery consists of seeing what everybody has seen, and thinking what nobody has thought".

Chapter 12

Conclusion

The most characteristic feature of glaucoma but rarely brought forward: the one million or so densely packed NFs in the ONH are being destroyed in an orderly sequence. This never occurs randomly.

Ironically, we don't take into account this most pathognomonic feature of glaucoma without which no glaucoma theory would be complete and valid. We have put forward various glaucoma theories ranging from corneal hysteresis to a brain disease without taking into account the orderly loss of NFs in glaucoma.

None of the prevalent glaucoma theories has attempted to incorporate the orderly loss of NFs – the most crucial aspect of glaucoma. Unless a glaucoma theory answers the question of orderly loss of NFs as well - it will be of no value.

Why are the NFs being destroyed, one-by-one, in an orderly sequence in glaucoma? This feat can't be accomplished by any direct ischemic or direct mechanical insult to the NFs of the ONH due to elevated IOP. Nevertheless, the elevated intraocular pressure is definitively the cause of glaucoma.

Furthermore, the glaucomatous field defects such as arcuate defects corroborate with the arrangement of NFs in the ONH suggesting that the ONH is the site of injury in glaucoma. We are faced with a big dilemma. How is elevated IOP causing orderly destruction of one million or so densely packed NFs of the optic disc?

In order to solve this mystery we have to take into consideration the three established facts of glaucoma.

First, without doubt, elevated IOP is definitively the cause of glaucoma. Second, the ONH is definitively the site of injury in glaucoma. Third, the nerve fibers are being destroyed in an orderly sequence, never randomly.

One thing is certain. If elevated IOP couldn't cause the orderly loss of NFs by its direct action or by any biological way, then the elevated IOP must be causing the orderly loss of NFs through some indirect and mechanical way. What could that mechanical scenario be?

I propose that glaucoma is a two-stage disease. The first stage, a biological stage: there is degeneration of the border tissue of Elschnig (BT) due to chronic ischemia induced either by elevated IOP - above 21mmHg or normal range IOP (below 21mmHg) but acting as elevated IOP.

Degeneration of the BT will result in sinking of the LC and initiation of the mechanical stage. The second, or mechanical stage in fact is the start of perimetric glaucoma which will result in the self-propagated orderly loss of NFs until all the NFs are severed.

For, one-by-one destruction, the NFs should be lying loose so they could be easily separated. This is only possible when the NFs are lying loose in the prelaminar area, not when the NFs are fastened into bundles in the intricate meshwork of the lamina cribrosa. Although it is widely believed, in view of the orderly loss of NFs, the LC couldn't be the site of injury in glaucoma.

There are two main aspects of my hypothesis. First, the LC is sinking in the scleral canal. Secondly, it is resulting in the stretching and severance of NFs. Sinking of the LC and severance of NFs are unique features of glaucoma, not seen in any other disease.

My hypothesis rejects the theories of cupping and the lamina cribrosa as the site of injury in glaucoma. The NFs are not being atrophied but severed. Glaucoma may not be an optic neuropathy as commonly believed, but an optic axotomy- a paradigm shift.

REFERENCES

1. Anderson, DR. Probing the Floor of the Optic Nerve Head in Glaucoma Ophthalmology 2012; 119:1-2.

2. Armaly MF Cup/disc ratio in early open-angle glaucoma. Doc Ophthalmol 1969;526-33

2. Concise Ophthalmology Text & Atlas Fifth Edition: Syed Imtiaz Ali Shah. Paramount Books, Karachi, Pakistan 2016.

3. Duke-Elder S, Barrie J. Diseases of the lens and vitreous, glaucoma and hypotony, System of Ophthalmology, Vol. X1. London: Henry Kimpton; 1969.

4. Eliesa Ing, et al. Cupping in the Monkey Optic Nerve Transection Model Consists of Prelaminar Tissue Thinning in the Absence of Posterior Laminar Deformation. Invest Ophthalmol Vis Sci. 2016; 57: 2598-2611.

5. Fortune, B., Reynaud, J., Hardin, C., Wang, L., Sigal, I. A., & Burgoyne, C. F. (2016). Experimental Glaucoma Causes Optic Nerve Head Neural Rim Tissue Compression: A Potentially Important Mechanism of Axon Injury. Investigative Ophthalmology & Visual Science, 57(10), 4403–4411. http://doi.org/10.1167/iovs.16-20000

6. Akram, Amjad et al. Glaucoma: Pearls for the Ophthalmic Resident. Paramount Books, Karachi, Pakistan.2015.

7. Harrington, D. Pathogenesis of Glaucomatous Visual Field Defects: Individual Variations in Pressure Sensitivity in Glaucoma. In Transactions of Fifth Macy Conference, 1960. Princeton , N.J., Josiah Macy, Jr. Foundation, 1961, p259

8. Hayreh SS. Structure and Blood Supply of the Optic Nerve. In: Heilmann K, Richardson KT, editors. Glaucoma: Conceptions of a Disease. Stuttgart: Theime; 1978.

9. Hasnain SS. Optic Disc may be Sinking in Chronic glaucoma. Ophthalmology Update. Oct-Dec. 2010; 8 (4); 22-28.

10. Hasnain SS. Scleral Edge, not Optic Disc or Retina is the Primary Site of Injury in Chronic Glaucoma. Medical Hypothesis 2006; 67(6); 1320-1325

11. Hasnain SS. Are Nerve Fibers being Atrophied or Severed in Glaucoma? Ophthalmology Update. Pakistan Oct-Dec 2013, 11(4) 226-228

12. Hasnain SS. Can Glaucoma be Can a Neurodegenerative Disease? Highlights of Ophthalmology. Panama 2012 40(3)

13. Hasnain SS. A Simple Method to Diagnose Glaucoma. Ophthalmology Update. Pakistan January-March 2013 11(1).

14. Hasnain SS. Pathogenesis of Arcuate Field Defects in Glaucoma. Highlights of Ophthalmology, Panama 2012 40(6)

15. Hasnain SS. The Missing Piece in Glaucoma? Open Journal of Ophthalmology 6: 56-62

16. Hasnain SS. Are We on Right Path in Glaucoma? Ophthalmology Update: Vol 12. No. 4, October – December 2014.

17. Hasnain SS. Pathogenesis of Orderly Loss of Nerve Fibers in Glaucoma: Optometry; Open Access, 2016, 1:2

18. Hayreh SS: Pathogenesis of Visual Field Defects: Role of Ciliary Circulation. British Journal of Ophthalmology, 54: 289, 1970

19. Henkind, P. (1967). Radial Peripapillary Capillaries of the Retina. I. Anatomy: Human and Comparative. British Journal of Ophthalmology, 51(2), 115–123.

20. Kuhn, Thomas S. (1970). The Structure of Scientific Revolutions. Chicago: University of Chicago Press.

21. Lee Km, et al. 2014. Anterior Lamina Cribrosa Insertion in Primary Open-Angle and Healthy Subjects. PLOS One 9(12).

22. Maumenee E: The Pathogenesis of Visual Field Loss in Glaucoma: Brockhurst RJ et al, (editors): Controversy in Ophthalmology. Philadelphia:WB Saunders Company;1977 p301-11.

23. Park SC et al. In-vivo, 3-Dimensional Imaging of the Lamina Cribrosa Horizontal Central Ridge in Normals and Lamina Cribrosa Deformation in Glaucoma. Investigative Ophthalmology and Visual Science. 2011; 52:3063.

24. Quigly HA, Addicks EM. Regional Differences in the Structure of the Lamina Cribrosa and their Relation to the Glaucomatous Optic Nerve Damage. Arch Ophthalmol 1981; 99:137-43

25. Sadun AA. Papilledema and Raised Intracranial Pressure. In: Yanoff M, Duker J, editors. Ophthalmology. London: Mosby; 1999.

26. Shields MB, Textbook of Glaucoma, 3rd ed. Baltimore, MD: Williams & Wilkens 1992: 515-516.

27. Wolff E. Anatomy of the Eye and Orbit Revised by Last, RJ. 6th Ed. London: H.K. Lewis & Co; 1968.

28. Yang H. et al. Posterior (Outward) Migration of the Lamina Cribrosa and Early Cupping in Monkey Experimental Glaucoma. Invest Ophthalmol Vis Sci 2011; 52:7109-21.

29. Yang H. Optic Nerve Head (ONH) Lamina Cribrosa Insertion Migration and Pialization in Early Non-Human Primate Experimental Glaucoma. Poster Presentation ARVO Meeting May 03, 2010.

30. Yanoff M, Fine BS. Ocular Pathology. Maryland: Harper & Row; 1975.

31. Yarmohammadi A et al. Optical Coherence Tomography Angiography Vessel Density in Healthy, Glaucoma Suspect, and Glaucoma Eyes. Invest Ophthalmol Vis Sci 2016 July.

32. Zeried FM, Osuagwu UL(2013) Changes in Retinal Nerve Fiber Layer and Optic Disc Algorithms by Optical Coherence Tomography in Glaucomatous Arab Subjects. Clinical Ophthalmology 7: 1941-1949.